Quantitative Explorations in Drug Abuse Policy

Quantitative Explorations in Drug Abuse Policy

Edited by
Irving Leveson
Director of Economic Studies
Hudson Institute
Croton-on-Hudson, New York

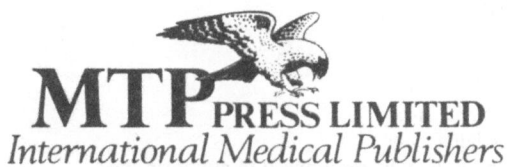

MTP PRESS LIMITED
International Medical Publishers

Published in the UK and Europe by
MTP Press Limited
Falcon House
Lancaster, England

Published in the US by
SPECTRUM PUBLICATIONS, INC.
175-20 Wexford Terrace
Jamaica, N.Y. 11432

ISBN-13:978-94-011-7717-7   e-ISBN-13:978-94-011-7715-3
DOI:10.1007/978-94-011-7715-3

Contributors

EDWARD B. BACHMAN, Ph.D.
Research Associate
Institute for Research in Social
  Science
University of North Carolina
Chapel Hill, North Carolina

GEORGE F. BROWN, JR., Ph.D.
Managing Consultant
Data Resources, Inc.
Washington, D.C.

DOUGLAS C. COATE, Ph.D.
Assistant Professor
Department of Economics
Rutgers University
Newark, New Jersey

ALVIN M. CRUZE, Ph.D.
Director
Center for the Study of Social
  Behavior
Research Triangle Institute
Reserch Triangle Park, North
  Carolina

LUCY N. FRIEDMAN, Ph.D.
Director
N.Y.C. Victims Services Agency
New York, New York

FRED GOLDMAN, Ph.D.
Assistant Professor of Public Health
School of Public Health
Columbia University
New York, New York

GLORIA A. GRIZZLE, Ph.D.
Associate Professor
Florida State University
Tallahassee, Florida

IRVING LEVESON, Ph.D.
Director of Economic Studies
Hudson Institute
Croton-on-Hudson, New York

J. VALLEY RACHAL, Ph.D.
Coordinator
Substance Abuse Programs
Center for the Study of Social
  Behavior
Research Triangle Institute
Research Triangle Park, North
  Carolina

BRENT L. RUFENER, Ph.D
Economist
Center for the Study of Social
  Behavior
Research Triangle Institute
Research Triangle Park, North
  Carolina

LESTER P. SILVERMAN, Ph.D.
Office of Policy Analysis
U.S. Department of the Interior
Washington, D.C.

EDUARDO N. SIGUEL, Ph.D.
Division of Scientific and Program
  Information
National Institute on Drug Abuse
Rockville, Maryland

ANN D. WITTE, Ph.D.
Associate Professor
Department of Economics
University of North Carolina
Chapel Hill, North Carolina

ACKNOWLEDGEMENTS

The skills and cooperation of each of the authors made this undertaking especially rewarding. Valuable comments were received from Lucy Friedman, Gloria Grizzle, Eduardo Siguel, Lester Silverman, and Ann Witte. The work benefited from early discussions with Anthony Jaffa and Heather Ruth. Special thanks are due to Fred Goldman for suggestions on the entire enterprise. The editor also wishes to express appreciation for the efforts of Wendy Asher and Anita Steinberg in editing and production and to Maurice Ancharoff, President of Spectrum Publications, for patience and continued support at formative stages.

Introduction

IRVING LEVESON

The 1960s was a period of rapid social and economic change, coupled with spectacular growth in the role of government in dealing with social issues. The demands of public programs and policies created enormous pressures for improved information and analyses. In the field of drug abuse these pressures were compounded by the rapid rise of drug use and the absence of much critical information and analysis. The most elementary steps to develop a data base were just beginning, and many years of effort would be required before the accumulation of knowledge could produce a strong foundation for public policy.

There has been enormous progress in improving knowledge about drug abuse since the mid-1960s. However, as in many fields, research has concentrated on a few questions while others largely are ignored, and even where studies exist there are problems of assimilation. Information is widely dispersed, not always accessible and often not in the most useful form. Many analysts do not have adequate understanding of the ways in which studies might enter into policy development, while at the same time, persons responsible for policy formation often do not have sufficient knowledge of how to use research to help resolve policy issues. A major objective of this volume is to illustrate the formation of linkages which may bridge the gap between research and policy.

The selections deal with problems in the areas of epidemiology and social cost, prevention, deterrence, education, treatment, employment and supportive services. For the most part the studies apply to heroin abuse. This is an outcome of the available state of quantitative research as well as the particular familiarity of the editor with these materials.

The first four chapters consider aspects of the measurement of addiction and its social costs. Rufener, Rachal, and Cruze develop detailed estimates of costs of drug abuse in the criminal justice system, addiction programs, medical care and lost productivity. The costs to society of drug abuse are estimated at between $8.4 and $12.2 billion in Fiscal Year 1975. Differences in methodology and findings from previous studies are examined. An important improvement in the methodology over other studies is that the crime attributed to drug abuse is measured by the additional crime committed by abusers rather than all crime by abusers, some of which might have been committed by the same individuals in the absence of drug abuse.[1] To make this distinction the authors rely on an early version of the study by Coate and Goldman in Chapter 4.

Coate and Goldman develop a model which enables them to estimate the effects of a one-dollar increase in drug expenditures on criminal earnings. The method depends on examining differences among individuals in size of habit. The analysis is carried out for a Phoenix House population of 998 persons in New York City. Coate and Goldman find, according to one estimate, that a dollar greater drug consumption leads to $.18-$.29 in additional earnings from general criminal activity. The remainder is financed by sales of drugs, legal earnings, transfer payments such as Public Assistance and other sources. Rufener, Rachal, and Cruze use a $.30 figure in their calculations. In the absence of additional information they extrapolate this share of drug costs from crime directly to a national population.[2]

Hunt and Chambers (1976) and Dupont and Greene (1973) have supplemented current indicators of drug abuse with historical series constructed from information on persons in treatment in selected cities. Year of first heroin use is determined from a population in treatment at a point in time and the data arranged to represent the number of new heroin abusers in each year. Time series

---

[1]Information on the effects of addiction on crime has been rather limited, although some good literature reviews exist. See Goldman and Coate (1977), Greenberg and Adler [n.d.] and Jacoby et al. (1973).

[2]Coate and Goldman also find that the share of drug costs made up of illegal earnings is greater for users of drugs other than heroin than it is for users of heroin. Since drugs other than heroin tend to cost less, this may mean that their debilitating effects were greater than heroin or that their heavy use was associated with less work-oriented life styles. Since the population studied was residing in a therapeutic community this also may reflect the selection of a group for which use of drugs other than heroin was particularly limiting or whose attachment to the labor force was particularly weak.

constructed from year of first use show peak use most typically occurring around 1969.

Several authors have criticized the method which Hunt and others use to infer timing (Richman and Abbey, 1976; Gould in Rittenhouse, 1976). The most important of their grounds for believing that a large bias may occur is that there is a delay between first use and admission to treatment. This delay could in theory cause the lag pattern to be mistaken for a pattern of changes in incidence over time. While Hunt and Chambers (1976, p. 110) make a correction for exclusion of those who have not entered treatment, there is no available series which satisfactorily adjusts for any tendency for the lag distribution to appear as if it is a fluctuation in incidence. The more important question, however, is whether an adjustment is really necessary.

Siguel (Chapter 2) attempts to separate the effects of incidence and lag distribution in data from a population in treatment for the entire United States. He compares population groups which have different lag distributions to determine if they have patterns of incidence with similar timing. There is a peak at about 1969 for groups having different lag distributions. This finding is consistent with the interpretation that the peak reflects the pattern of incidence. (In some cases there is a secondary peak which may be produced by the lag in entry into treatment.)

Siguel's extensive data, much in the form of unpublished tables, offer a still more powerful refutation of the notion that the 1969 peak is an artifact of the lag distribution. Suppose the lag in the earlier analyses of the 1972 admission cohort had produced a 1969 peak as a statistical artifact. If the lag in entry into treatment remained constant, for persons admitted to treatment in 1975, the peak should have occurred three years earlier in 1972. Yet Siguel's charts show that peak incidence in Washington, D.C. continues to be around 1969 for persons admitted to treatment in 1975 and 1976. There is no evidence that a corresponding increase occurred in the lag in entry into treatment. These, and similar findings for New York and other cities, clearly imply that the 1969 data for the peak in year of first heroin use is real.

When the price of heroin rises, drug users do not have as much of an opportunity to adjust legal sources of income in the short run as they would over a longer period of time. While some may reduce size of habit, the number of users would not be expected to decrease to the same degree as if the price of heroin remained high for a long time. Brown and Silverman (Chapter 3) construct a time series of heroin prices adjusted for purity and size of buy on a monthly basis from 1970 to 1972. When the price series is used to estimate the response of crime to fluctuations in heroin price in New York City, they find that a 10 percent increase in price is associated with an increase of 1.4 to 3.6 percent in property crime in various categories. These short-run responses can be translated into an approximate measure of the proportion of crime committed by addicts. They suggest a magnitude of 14 to 36 percent or approximately 23 percent as an average for all crimes. Leveson (Chapter 5) estimates the proportion at the lower end of this range.

While there is a positive association between crime and the price of heroin for New York, the results for other cities are mixed. In a companion study, Silverman and Spruill (1977) found strong evidence for Detroit as well. The prospect that crime would increase after a rise in the price of heroin following increased enforcement has at times been a deterrent to police action.

Chapters 5 through 7 deal with various aspects of the determinants of the quantity of drug abuse and the number of abusers. Leveson (Chapter 5) examines interstate differences in opiate-use rates in 1961 in a multivariate analysis. The demand analysis found a statistically significant relationship of drug use to race and to poverty, defined as the proportion of families with income below half a state's median income. Median family income had a very strong positive effect on opiate-use rates after controlling for other variables. This suggests that income growth could produce substantial increases in drug use over time.

In Chapter 6, Leveson compares changes over time in indicators of heroin incidence and prevalence with other developments which may explain the variations observed. Exploratory comparisons suggest that changing international supplies have played a dominant role in the changing rates of heroin use. These factors include not only the off-and-on effects of the Turkish opium ban and the growth in supplies from Mexico, but also fluctuations which appear to be associated with the rise and decline of commerce to Southeast Asia in the Vietnam era. The hypothesis that shifts in supply dominated the movements in heroin indicators is supported by comparisons of directions of movement of price and quantity series. The behavior of several socioeconomic variables in the United States is also considered and some speculations offered about their role. Youth unemployment is suggested as a particularly promising subject for further research.

In recent years there has been a substantial accumulation of evidence that the prospects for punishment and the size of the expected penalty exert a strong influence on the amount of criminal behavior in a population. Such findings cannot be applied mechanically in estimating addict responses. The addiction itself may lead to smaller or slower changes. Furthermore, increases in enforcement tend to raise the price of heroin. Addicts may steal more in order to meet the higher prices and this effect may lead to even greater crime. The issue becomes even more complex when it is broken down into questions of enforcement against various drugs, at various levels of the distribution system and through alternative programmatic instruments (see Moore, 1977).

General law enforcement would be expected to have particularly strong effects on addiction if the criminal justice system treated addicts and nonaddicts unequally. There are indications that in New York City (Manhattan) addicts have higher probabilities of pretrial detention than others (Sajovic, 1975, p. 18-20). This suggests that in addition to general effects the criminal justice system may act much like an involuntary incarceration program.

One use of information on the effects of penalties is in determining the effect of legal status on the social costs of drug use. While legalization would increase the number of drug abusers, it would greatly lower the cost of the drugs and the associated crime per use. The social costs would rise only if the number of users expanded proportionally more than the crime and other social costs per user fell. While reasonable assumptions could be made about the degree to which social costs per user would fall, there is still no acceptable way to gauge the prospective expansion in the number of users.

Leveson (Chapter 5) presents three tests of enforcement effects: 1) A crude test of crossover effects in an interstate analysis finds no relationship between penalties for marijuana possession and use of opiates. 2) Time series analysis suggests a definite negative relationship between drug arrests and narcotic-related deaths over time in New York City prior to the rapid growth of addiction. Thereafter the growth itself causes the two indicators to rise together. 3) Tests across states in 1961 provide no evidence that the reported number of opiate users is lower, other things being equal, in states with a high probability of punishment for major crimes generally. The interstate comparisons rely on the probability of punishment for all offenses rather than drug offenses alone.

Aggregate data do not clearly distinguish between enforcement against users and enforcement against distributors. This distinction is of course blurred because many users are small distributors. In an analysis of individual behavior, Bachman and Witte (Chapter 7) examine a sample of male North Carolina prisoners following release. Bachman and Witte use the individual's length of sentence as a measure of his expected penalty for further crime. They find that a greater length of sentence is associated with fewer post-release arrests for both ex-addicts and others. However, perverse effects are found when the strength of deterrence was measured by the individual's expected probability of arrest and conviction.

Supervision is found to decrease the frequency of post-release arrest. Parole appears to be particularly effective in deterring ex-addicts, in comparison with alcoholics and other offenders. A related issue is the question of the role of compulsion in the success of treatment programs. The New York State program of involuntary incarceration was unsuccessful because of high cost, high abscondance rates, and high recidivism (Chapter 9). However, compulsion may be an important element when properly used. The strong effects of surveillance in a post-prison release population found by Bachman and Witte are not the only evidence pointing in this direction. The Washington, D.C. court diversion program showed gains when persons were continuously monitored after being referred to treatment. Sheffet et al. (1975) found much higher retention rates in a therapeutic community in the face of legal pressure.

Bachman and Witte provide an interesting test of the effects of income maintenance. They find that prisoners who were able to accumulate the greatest amount of work release earnings had the greatest likelihood of rearrest after release from prison, presumably as a result of more rapid return to drugs. However, the analysis also suggests that the adverse effects did not occur when surveillance was also provided.

Most evidence relates to persons who have been using drugs for some time. However, there is reason to believe the effects of deterrence are much greater for new or potential users than others. The tendency for drugs to be distributed free to encourage first use is one indication that making use less costly has a relatively large impact (Moore, 1973). Another indication is the relatively greater contagion effects for new users found by Hunt and Chambers (1976). Other indications come from evidence of strong responsiveness of youth to incentive factors in studies of migration and labor market behavior. The material in Chapter 6 is not inconsistent with this interpretation.

Chapters 8 through 10 deal with the effectiveness of education, treatment and supportive service programs. If young persons respond more readily to various stimuli, a properly designed drug education program might be expected to have a large effect. Grizzle's examination of the effects of a program in Charlotte, North Carolina between 1972 and 1974 is reported in Chapter 8. Behavior of approximately 24,000 students in 14 "experimental" and 12 "non-experimental" schools is compared to determine the impact of the program on usage of a variety of drugs, on drug knowledge and on the percentage of students in high-risk psychological states. Grizzle finds important effects of drug education on usage for the program studied.

There has been increasing concern that when drug education programs raise student interest and provide greater knowledge of drugs they tend to increase rather than decrease drug use (Wald et al., 1972). Grizzle finds no evidence to support this view, but she also notes that the program emphasis changed when the possibility of such effects became a matter of concern.

Education is particularly difficult to evaluate because the content and quality of programs can vary enormously. The careful efforts of this study provide confidence in the findings for this program but leave uncertain how much the results can be generalized.

While a variety of treatment methods have evolved to deal with the problem of drug abuse, knowledge of the effectiveness of alternative treatments remain limited. The need to vary treatments with circumstances creates demands for information not only on details such as dosage responses but also on broad issues of the appropriateness of treatment approaches for different population groups. Where experimental variation is not possible it becomes necessary to use statistical techniques to infer what would happen if treatments varied. Leveson (Chapter 9) considers the problem of matching treatments and patients based on aggregate data.

A central part of the analysis consists of an examination of the "maturation hypothesis" which states that addicts tend to mature out of addiction after a period of years. The age distributions of persons reported to the New York City Narcotics Register, together with assumptions about maturation, imply a pattern of growth of addiction in the past. The age distributions are found to be consistent with some form of maturation since, if maturation did not occur, unreasonable patterns of growth of addiction over time would be implied.

Because of maturing out of addiction, the length of time a person can be expected to continue abusing drugs varies with age. Differences among persons of different ages in the remaining number of years of addiction must be taken into account in calculating benefits of treatment programs.[3] The approach suggests, for example, that it might be beneficial for methadone programs to admit persons below age 20 even though the retention rates are low, since the benefits would be collected for a longer period than for older persons.

To date, the most significant attempt to provide employment for former drug abusers, together with treatment and other services, is the Wildcat program in New York City. The evaluation of that program, which is summarized in Chapter 10, led to the expansion of supported employment on a national scale. Friedman (Chapter 10) finds that the benefits do exceed the costs, but not dramatically. Furthermore, it was exceedingly difficult to identify which persons would have done well without supported employment. The study also found that there were important benefits in reduced public assistance payments and that female former abusers had greater problems in finding and holding jobs than males.

When I first became interested in drug abuse research in 1967, I was impressed most by the dogmatism of many discussions of drug abuse policy and of the absence of processes to assure objective research. Since that time, work in the field has come a long way. The contributions to this volume illustrate only a part of the growing literature which is both making the criteria for policy decisions explicit and providing a factual foundation on which intelligent choices can be based.

---

[3]Application of the suggested measure of effectiveness to an extensive set of comparisons among policies and programs can be found in Leslie (1976). This approach was also reached by Grizzle in Chapter 8.

LEVESON

REFERENCES

Dupont, Robert and Greene, Mark, "The dynamics of a heroin addiction epidemic," *Science,* 181 (August 24, 1973), pp. 716-722.

Goldman, Fred and Coate, Douglas, "The Relationship Between Drug Addiction and Participation in Criminal Activities," unpublished manuscript, Columbia University School of Public Health, June 1975.

Greenberg, Stephanie and Adler, Frieda, *Crime and Addiction, An Empirical Analysis of the Literature, 1920-1973,* Report Series Number One, Governor's Council on Drug and Alcohol Abuse, State of Pennsylvania (nid).

Hunt, Leon and Chambers, Carl, *The Heroin Epidemics, A Study of Heroin Use in the United States, 1965-1975,* New York: Spectrum Publications, Inc., 1976.

Jacoby, Joseph E., Weiner, Neil A., Thornbeny, Terence P., and Wolfgang, Marvin, "Drug use and criminality in a birth cohort," in National Commission on Marijuana and Drug Abuse, *Drug Abuse in America, Appendix,* Volume 1: *Patterns and Consequences of Drug Use,* Washington: U.S. Government Printing Office, 1973, pp. 300-345.

Leslie, Allan, "Benefit-cost analysis of New York City heroin addiction problems and programs-1971," *Analysis of Urban Health Problems,* edited by Irving Leveson and Jeffrey Weiss, New York: Spectrum Publications, Inc., 1976, pp. 112-137.

Moore, Mark, *Buy and Bust,* Lexington, Mass.: Lexington Books, 1977.

Moore, Mark, "Policies to achieve discrimination on the effective price of heroin," *American Economic Review,* 63, No. 2 (May, 1973), pp. 270-277.

Richman, Alex and Abbey, Helen, "Heroin epidemics—the decline and fall of epidemiologic research," *Proceedings of the Social Statistics Section of the American Statistical Association, 1976,* Part II, pp. 711-716.

Rittenhouse, Joan Dunne (editor), *Report of the Task Force on The Epidemiology of Heroin and Other Narcotics,* Stanford, Calif.: Stanford Research Institute, December, 1976.

Sajovic, Majda, "Crime committed by narcotics users in Manhattan," Drug Law Evaluation Project of the Association of the Bar of the City of New York, May, 1976.

Sheffet, A.M., Quinonies, M., Lavenhar, M.A., Nakah, A., Prager, H., Doyle, K., and Louria, D., "Extra-mural evaluation of drug addiction treatment programs," paper presented at the Annual Meeting of the American Public Health Association, November, 1975.

Silverman, Lester P., and Spruill, Nancy C., "Urban crime and the price of heroin," *Journal of Urban Economics,* 4 (1977), pp. 80-103.

Wald, Patricia, et al., *Dealing with Drug Abuse,* New York: Praeger Publishers, 1972.

Quantitative Explorations in Drug Abuse Policy

Contents

CHAPTER 1

Costs of Drug Abuse to Society

BRENT L. RUFENER
J. VALLEY RACHAL
ALVIN M. CRUZE

This chapter provides an estimate of the total economic costs experienced by society in the 1975 fiscal year due to the abuse of drugs. These costs have been developed from existing secondary data sources and from the latest research findings concerning the extent of drug abuse in the United States and the association between drug abuse and other forms of behavior that impose costs to society. In addition, the results of this study build on previous efforts to estimate these costs, most notably studies by A.D. Little (1974) and Johns Hopkins (Lemkau et al., 1975).

This study does not purport to be the definitive answer regarding the economic costs to society of drug abuse. In some cases it was necessary to use data of questionable reliability where nothing better was available. In other cases it was necessary to use data from small, limited studies to estimate totals for the entire United States. For some cost components, too little is known about the related behavioral phenomena to provide definitive conclusions regarding the impact of drug abuse. For example, the amount of nondrug criminal activity "caused" by drug abuse is an important question about which definite answers are not yet available. Subject to the qualifications given, we feel, however, that this study presents a useful national estimate of the economic costs to society of drug abuse in fiscal year 1975.

1

In conducting a cost analysis of this nature, a useful initial step is an enumeration of all the costs that will be borne by society. This initial step can be thought of as developing a cost framework or model and is undertaken in order to ensure the inclusion of all relevant costs. Obviously, if some cost items are left out the total cost will be understated; if costs that are not relevant are included, total costs will be overstated. Thus, the cost framework itself as well as measurement of each individual cost item is fundamentally important.

The total economic cost of drug abuse is derived by separately estimating the various cost components. In order to develop the cost estimates it was necessary to make a number of assumptions. Among the most critical was an assumption concerning the number of drug abusers in the U.S. Three assumptions were made concerning the number of heroin addicts—250,000 500,000, and 750,000—with three resulting estimates of the costs of drug abuse.

Based on the framework and assumptions developed in this study, the economic costs to society of drug abuse for fiscal year 1975 are estimated to be

Table 1. The Economic Costs of Drug Abuse
Fiscal Year 1975
($ Millions)

Cost Component	Assumed Number of Addicts*		
	Low	Middle	High
Direct Costs	$4,265	$4,932	$5,599
Medical Expenses	494	494	494
Law Enforcement	1,342	1,342	1,342
Judicial System	296	296	296
Correction	294	294	294
Nondrug Crime	667	667	667
Drug Traffic Control	93	93	93
Drug Abuse Prevention	995	995	995
Housing Stock Loss	84	84	84
Indirect Costs	$4,167	$5,406	$6,644
Unemployability	1,239	2,478	3,716
Emergency Room Treatment	0.4	0.4	0.4
Inpatient Hospitalization	20	20	20
Mental Hospitalization	8	8	8
Drug-related Deaths	12.5	12.5	12.5
Absenteeism	1,594	1,594	1,594
Incarceration	1,205	1,205	1,205
Treatment Costs	88	88	88
TOTAL COSTS	$8,432	$10,338	$12,243

*The assumed numbers of addicts were: 250,000; 500,000; and 750,000.

between $8.4 and $12.2 billion, with a middle estimate of $10.3 billion. Approximately 48 percent of these costs are due to direct costs or expenditures for services or goods needed as a direct result of drug abuse. The remaining portion of the total costs are indirect costs and result from decreased production of goods and services as a result of drug abuse. The sizes of the components which enter into these calculations are shown in Table 1 and Figure 1.

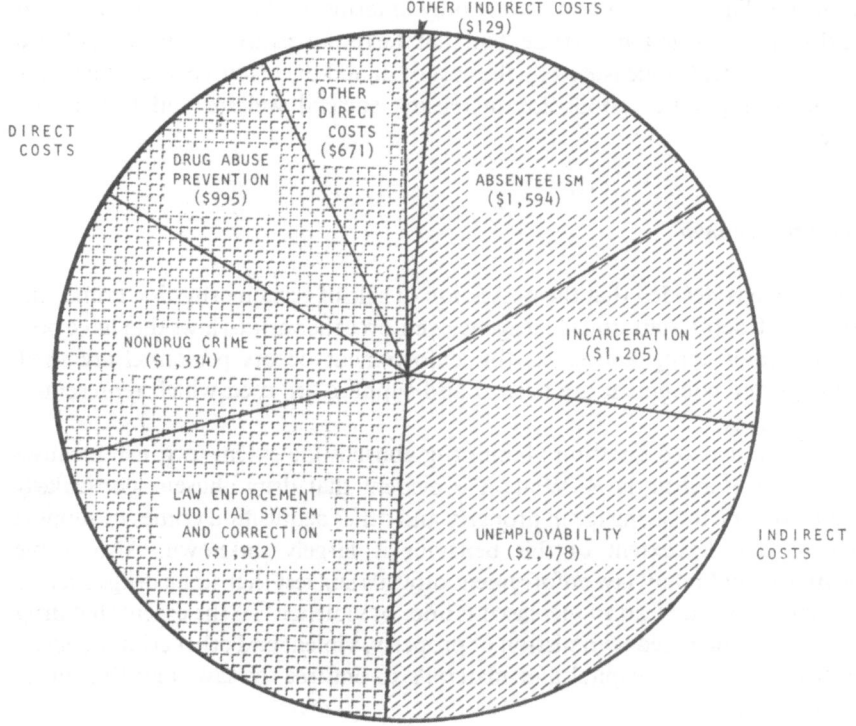

Fig. 1. Components of the Economic Costs of Drug Abuse, Fiscal Year 1975 ($ Millions).

COST COMPONENTS

Brief explanations of the direct and indirect cost components other than medical care may make clearer the meaning of these figures:

Direct Costs

Direct costs are estimated in terms of expenditures required for the component because of drug abuse; however, from a somewhat more economic, theoretic point of view these costs represent use of scarce resources for producing the service indicated, a service which in the absence of drug abuse would not be produced. This is of value to society only in terms of alleviating some aspect of the drug abuse problem. To the extent that the resources are used because of drug abuse (the extent is measured by the cost estimate) the resources are unavailable for producing other goods for increasing societal welfare and thus a cost is incurred.

Law Enforcement

Society has decided that the possession or sale of certain drugs is a crime, and therefore, federal, state and local agencies enforce the various laws that have been passed against drug abuse. As this enforcement occurs personnel are used, buildings and equipment are needed and supplies are used which represents a cost to society.

A widely debated question about drug abuse is the extent to which it causes violation of nondrug laws. While it is evident that drug abusers, particularly heroin abusers, must engage in property and other acquisition crimes to support their habits, the extent of this behavior is largely unknown. Also, some researchers and many law enforcement officials suggest that some drugs such as the stimulants may lead to increased crimes of violence. To the extent that drug abuse causes increased commission of property, violent and other crimes, society will use more labor, capital and materials to enforce the laws and thus incur resource costs.

Judicial System

As violators of drug and nondrug laws are arrested and processed through the criminal justice system personnel are used in staffing courts, prosecution and defense; buildings and equipment are used; and supplies are used. All of these resource uses are a cost to society.

Corrections

Some of those convicted of violation of drug laws and nondrug laws will be incarcerated, and others will be placed on probation. Obviously, for those convicted of violation of drugs laws the resource costs for correction are related to drug abuse; for violators of nondrug laws we again must assume a relationship between criminal behavior and drug abuse.

Nondrug Crime

Becker (1968) and Tullock (1967) indicated that the total real income loss to society from crime is the sum of (a) the labor and capital inputs into criminal activity and (b) the costs of controlling crime. This latter cost, which consists of enforcement, judicial system, and correction costs was discussed above. The labor and capital inputs into criminal activity represent a cost to society in that the resources used for criminal activities are unavailable for other uses. The amount of labor and capital used in criminal activities is a direct cost because as this resource is used it is paid with stolen goods (payment in kind) and/or stolen cash. Several analyses of the social costs of drug abuse refer to the value of stolen property as the direct cost of drug abuse. In fact, however, it is only an indirect measure of the labor and capital inputs to criminal activity. The value of the stolen goods contains an involuntary transfer element which is not a cost to society. Including this involuntary transfer as part of the costs of nondrug crime (as many estimates have) grossly overestimates the social cost due to this component.

Drug Traffic Control

A number of federal agencies outside of the Justice Department (the costs of which were included in the enforcement component) use labor, equipment, buildings and supplies to attempt to control drug trafficking.

Drug Abuse Prevention

Society uses its resources to treat drug abusers, to educate the population, to train drug abuse personnel, to conduct research and evaluation, and to provide management and support.

Housing Stock Loss

This cost, which is associated with heroin abuse, occurs as addicts occupy vacant apartments as havens for heroin use and inadvertently start fires.

Indirect Costs

Indirect costs are a loss to society of goods and services that would have been produced if individuals had not been engaged in drug abusing activities. These costs are measured in this study in terms of foregone earnings. The basic assumption in using this technique is that the earnings measures used accurately estimate the actual goods and services that are not produced as a result of abusers being unavailable for work; it is further assumed that being unavailable for work is causally related to the drug usage.

Unemployability

In computing this cost component it is assumed that drug abuse results in higher levels of unemployment among abusers than would be the case in the absence of drug usage.

Drug-related Deaths

Drug abuse results in the premature death of some abusers. By dying prematurely society must forego the goods and services that could have been produced. The death of a producer is also the death of a consumer. However, the deduction of consumption would be incorrect since it is the costs to society that are being estimated. See U.S. Department of HEW [1976].

Absenteeism

Drug abuse not only results in lower levels of employment, but also, for those employed, in higher levels of absenteeism from the job. Thus, costs are incurred as production opportunities are foregone.

Incarceration

Abusers who are incarcerated for violations of drug laws or nondrug laws are not available for work and total societal production is thus decreased.

Work Lost Due to Treatment

Certain drug abuse treatment modalities do not allow clients to work while in treatment.

DISCUSSION

Given these cost estimates, it is possible to develop a more detailed examination of the various cost components and to indicate a number of general policy implications of the results of this study. These elements include a separation of costs into those associated with heroin abuse and those associated with other drugs, a detailed comparison of the costs of drug abuse as presented in this study with costs previously estimated in the A.D. Little and Hopkins studies, and a comparison of the costs of drug abuse with the costs of alcohol abuse and alcoholism to society. Each of these topics is briefly summarized as follows:

Costs of Heroin Abuse

The total estimated costs of drug abuse are the result of the abuse of many different types of drugs. It is possible to separate the costs into two major categories: (1) those due to heroin abuse and (2) those due to the abuse of other drugs. Based on the three assumptions concerning the number of heroin addicts, the estimates of the cost of heroin abuse range from $4.5 to 8.3 billion, with a median estimate of $6.4 billion. On the basis of this middle estimate, 62 percent of the total economic cost of drug abuse in fiscal year 1975 can be attributed to heroin abuse.

Comparison with Previous Studies

The two previous major efforts to develop estimates of the cost of drug abuse to society resulted in totals close to the one reported herein. The Hopkins study total cost of May 1975 was $10.904 billion and the Little study total cost of December 1974 was $9.749 billion. It is perhaps important to point out, however, that significant differences exist in the components assumed to arrive at these totals, as indicated by Table 2. The theoretical and operational reasons for these differences are developed in Appendices A and B of the full report and are not detailed here. A brief discussion of the reasons for the primary differences between the RTI (Research Triangle Institute) cost estimates and the estimates of the other two studies follows. Throughout this discussion, it should be noted that references to costs in the RTI study are for the middle estimate of the number of addicts.

The costs of medical expenses are higher in the RTI study due to the inclusion of the estimated number of inpatient episodes in the entire United States and the estimation of some miscellaneous medical expenses. Law enforcement, judicial system, and correction costs are lower in this study than in the Hopkins study because we have used an estimate of the extent of causality between drug abuse and crime, whereas the Hopkins study used a method which showed only an association. The totals for nondrug crime are of similar size in the Hopkins and RTI studies even though they were computed using different methods. The Hopkins study estimated this cost with unadjusted data that showed only an association between drug abuse and criminal behavior. This procedure over-estimates the amount of nondrug crime caused by abuse and leads to an overstatement of the cost. The Hopkins study also estimated this cost component by using the average dollar loss per offense. This overstates the cost to society since the dollar loss figures contain an involuntary transfer element that is a loss to the victim of the crime but a gain to the person buying the stolen goods. Thus, the involuntary transfer element represents zero net real costs when considering society as a whole.

The Little study estimated this cost component by using a common method of making assumptions about the number of addicts, the daily habit cost, the number of days at risk, and a fence factor. This procedure overstates the economic cost because the involuntary transfer element is included and because of severe distortions in the market for heroin. This study presents an estimate of these costs that can be more readily justified on the basis of economic theory, since we have attempted to measure the value of the labor and capital used in nondrug crime caused by drug abuse, which is a more appropriate measure of the real economic loss to society.

Turning to the indirect costs of drug abuse, the unemployability cost estimate in this study is higher than that of the other studies because of the assumption of a larger estimate of the foregone earnings of addicts. The inpatient hospitalization costs are higher in this study because the estimated inpatient episodes in the U.S. were used and because of the higher earnings figure.

Drug-related death costs were smaller in this study than in the Little study because we have estimated this cost component for only one year, whereas the

Table 2. The Economic Costs of Drug Abuse, by Summary Categories from Three Studies

Category	Little Study (12/74) $Mn	%	Hopkins Study (5/75) $Mn	%	RTI Study (5/76) $Mn	%
Direct Costs						
Medical Expenses	199.1	2.0	41.4	0.4	494	4.8
Law Enforcement	401.5	4.1	3,379.6	31.0	1,342	13.0
Judicial System	52.2	0.5	596.4	5.5	296	2.9
Correction	165.8	1.7	2,132.0	19.6	294	2.8
Nondrug Crime	6,300.0	64.6	1,121.4	10.3	1,334	12.9
Drug Traffic Control	254.7	2.6	98.6	0.9	93	0.9
Drug Abuse Prevention	849.4	8.7	670.4	6.1	995	9.6
Housing Stock Loss	*		*		84	0.8
Indirect Costs						
Unemployability	970.9	10.0	1,803.8	16.5	2,478	24.0
Emergency Room Treatment	*		*		0.4	-
Inpatient Hospitalization	8.2	-	0.9		20	0.2
Mental Hospitalization	*		3.1		8	-
Drug-related Deaths	267.4	2.7	4.2		12.5	0.1
Absenteeism	280.0	2.9	448.0	4.1	1,594	15.4
Incarceration	*		604.0	5.5	1,205	11.6
Treatment Costs	*		*		88	0.8
TOTAL	$9,749	100.0%	$10,904	100.0%	$10,338	100.0%

*Cost not computed.

Little study reported the total present value of lost earnings of those who died in one year. Absenteeism costs are larger in this study due to the inclusion of the estimated costs of absenteeism in the female labor force. This study has also included an estimate of the costs of incarceration for the entire U.S. whereas the Hopkins study estimated this cost only for 20 states. The different earnings figures used in the two studies also accounts for some of the difference.

Comparison With Costs of Other Social Problems

Finally, it may be useful to compare the economic costs of drug abuse to the costs of other social problems in order to gain some insight into the relative magnitude of the costs of these problems.

The economic costs of alcohol abuse and alcoholism are detailed in Table 3. We have not critically examined the cost data provided. Since the study estimated the costs in 1971 we are unable to precisely determine what the costs were in fiscal year 1975. However, we did adjust these costs using changes in

Table 3. Economic Costs of Alcohol Abuse and Alcoholism (Billions of Dollars)

Cost Component	1971 Prices	FY 1975 Prices*
Lost Production	$9.35	$11.98
Health and Medical	8.29	10.34
Motor Vehicle Accidents	6.44	8.25
Alcohol Programs and Research	0.64	0.82
Criminal Justice System	0.51	0.65
TOTAL	$25.23	$32.04

*Adjusted using the Consumer Price Index. For health and medical care the medical care group was used; for the other cost components the entire CPI less medical care was used.
SOURCE: Ralph Berry, James Boland, Joan Laxson, Donal Haylor and Margery Sillman, *The Economic Cost of Alcohol Abuse and Alcoholism* (Boston: Policy Analysis, Inc., 1974).

the Consumer Price Index over this four year period with an estimate of $32.04 billion.

SUMMARY

In summary, we believe the techniques used for developing the costs in this report are economically sound. The basic shortcomings of the estimates developed are related to the unavailability or deficiencies of the data used and/or of knowledge about relationships between drug abuse and behavioral or other phenomena. This is particularly true and relevant with respect to the criminal behavior/drug abuse and unemployment/drug abuse relationships, as mentioned previously. Further, we did not undertake to develop new and perhaps more appropriate data sources. The data used were for the most part developed for other uses; more appropriate data for the purpose at hand could probably be developed for several cost categories. We should also like to remind the reader that we attempted as a matter of practicality to deal only with tangible costs in this volume. We, and others, recognize the intangible costs, including those under the rubric "pain and suffering," as well as others such as neighborhood deterioration, official corruption, and tax base losses are probably extensive. Thus, in actuality the total economic costs due to drug abuse are probably underestimated. We think, however, that the data assembled and costs estimated can provide useful inputs for social policy.

ACKNOWLEDGMENTS

This chapter is exerpted from Brent L. Rufener, J. Valley Rachal and Alvin M. Cruze, *Management Effectiveness Measures for NIDA Drug Abuse Treatment Programs, Volume II: Costs to Society of Drug Abuse,* Research Triangle Park, N.C.: Research Triangle Institute, May, 1976. The research was sponsored by the National Institute on Drug Abuse under terms of Contract No. 271-75-1016.

REFERENCES

A.D. Little Co. *Social Cost of Drug Abuse.* Cambridge: A.D. Little Co., 1975. Draft copy.
Barton, William A. *DAWN, An Operational Analysis and Evaluation.* Rockville, Md.: Strategic Intelligence Staff, Office of Intelligence, National Institute on Drug Abuse, November 5, 1974. Draft copy.
Becker, Gary S. "Crime and punishment: An economic approach," *Journal of Political Economy* 76 (March/April 1968): pp. 169-217.
Fujii, Edwin T. "Public investment in the rehabilitation of heroin addicts," *Social Science*

Quarterly 55 (June 1974): pp. 49-50.

Glenn, William A. and Hartwell, Tyler D. *Review of Methods of Estimating Number of Narcotic Addicts.* Research Triangle Park, N.C.: Research Triangle Institute, August 1975.

Goldman, Fred. *The Relationship Between Drug Addiction and Participation in Criminal Activities: An Econometric Analysis.* New York: Center for Policy Research and Columbia University, 1975. Draft copy. The final version of this study appears in this volume.

Gould, Leroy C. "Crime and the addict: Beyond common sense." In *Drugs and the Criminal Justice System,* edited by James A. Inciardi and Carl D. Chambers. Beverly Hills: Sage Publications, 1974, pp. 57-76.

Greenberg, Stephanie W. and Adler, Freda, "Crime and addiction, an empirical analysis of the literature 1920-1973," *Contemporary Drug Problems* 3 (1974): pp. 221-270.

Lemkau, Paul V., Amsel, Zili, Sanders, Bruce, Amsel, Jonathan, and Seif, Thomas F. *Social and Economic Costs of Drug Abuse,* Contract No. 271-75-1021. Baltimore, Md.: Department of Mental Hygiene, School of Hygiene and Public Health, The Johns Hopkins University, May 1974.

Leslie, Alan C. *A Benefit/Cost Analysis of New York City's Heroin Addiction Problems and Programs, 1971.* New York: City of New York, Office of Program Analysis, Health Services Administration, 1972, reprinted in Irving Leveson and Jeffrey Weiss (eds.), *Analysis of Urban Health Problems,* New York: Spectrum Publications, Inc., 1976.

McGlothlin, William H. and Tabbush, Victor C. "Costs, benefits, and potential for alternative approaches to opiate addiction control." In *Drugs and the Criminal Justice System,* edited by James A. Inciardi and Carl D. Chambers. Beverly Hills: Sage Publications, 1974, pp. 77-124.

Moore, Mark. *Policy Concerning Drug Abuse in New York State, Vol. 3, The Economics of Heroin Distribution.* Croton-on-Hudson, N.Y.: Hudson Institute, 1970.

Stoloff, Peter, Levine, Daniel, and Spruill, Nancy. *Public Drug Treatment and Addict Crime.* Arlington, Va.: Public Research Institute, 1974.

Tullock, Gordon. "The welfare costs of tariffs, monopolies, and thefts," *Western Economic Journal* 5 (June 1967): pp. 224-233.

U.S. Department of Health, Education and Welfare, National Institute of Mental Health. *The Cost of Mental Illness-1971* by Daniel S. Levine and Dianne R. Levine. DHEW Publication No. (ADM) 76-265. Washington: U.S. Government Printing Office, 1975.

U.S. Department of health, Education and Welfare, Social Security Administration, "The economic cost of illness revisited" by Barbara S. Cooper and Doprothy P. Rice, in *Social Security Bulletin* 39:2, pp. 21-36. Washington: U.S. Government Printing Office, 1976.

CHAPTER 2

Incidence of Heroin Use For Voluntary And Involuntary Admissions to Treatment

EDUARDO N. SIGUEL*

The distribution of an admission cohort (clients admitted during a given period of time) according to year of first use depends on the incidence for the various years and the waiting time (lag) to enter treatment. Peaks in the distribution of admissions can be due to incidence peaks or peaks in the waiting time distribution. Using groups of daily heroin users who share a common incidence distribution but who have different waiting times to enter treatment it is possible to separate the effects due to incidence from those due to waiting time. In this paper, voluntary heroin admissions, involuntary admissions, and admissions from individuals in prison are used to plot the distribution of the admission cohort (for 1975) by year of first use. Clients are further divided into two categories: those with no prior treatment experiences and those with one or more, for a total of six mutually exclusive and exhaustive groups. It is shown that all groups share a common peak, attributed to incidence, in 1969. The peaks of the waiting time distributions for those with no prior experiences are seen to be around two to three years.

---

*The views presented in this paper do not necessarily represent the policies and opinions of the National Institute on Drug Abuse.

The methodology presented here supports the view that an epidemic of heroin use occurred in 1969, answers criticisms regarding the use of admission data for incidence studies, and suggests that incidence of heroin use increased in 1974.

The spread of heroin use from 1950 through the 1960s has been described as an epidemic phenomenon, a rapid increase in incidence (number of new heroin users in a given period of time). It has been difficult, however, to measure the trends in the incidence of heroin use because the data have been severely limited and controversial. Some of the indirect measures of incidence are the number of cases of serum hepatitus, overdose deaths, and the detection of heroin-positive urine specimens in an arrestee population. The number of serum hepatitus cases was used in earlier studies to outline the spread of heroin use to medium-sized cities and the same indicator was used to show a tenfold increase in heroin incidence from 1966 to 1972 in Washington, D.C. and the nation as a whole (Greene et al., 1974; Minichiello and Retka, 1976). Overdose death due to heroin use was the criterion employed to determine upward trends in the 1960s and a downward trend after 1969 (Ipsen et al., 1973; Huber et al., 1977; Greene and Dupont, 1974). The reduction in the number of urine-positive tests since 1971 was interpreted as indicating a downward trend in new heroin use (Greene and Dupont, 1974). Field observations and interview techniques were employed to detect trends in the incidence of heroin use in small geographical areas. Results from this methodology were used to infer the large spread of heroin use in the late 1960s in the areas investigated (De Alarcon, 1969; Hughes and Crawford, 1972; Levengood et al., 1973).

Of a more direct but somewhat controversial nature, the reported year of first heroin use (onset) by clients in an admission cohort (those who entered treatment within a given time period) has been used to make inferences about trends in incidence. This approach plots the distribution of the admissions according to each year of first use in order to obtain a curve which attempts to measure and visually depict incidence trends. Using this method, an epidemic, in the late 1960s, which peaked in 1969, was described for Washington, D.C.; another, which peaked about 1969 or 1970, was shown in the San Francisco Bay area; and a third epidemic of heroin use after World War II, which peaked about 1950, was described for the USA (Dupont and Greene, 1973; Newmeyer, 1974; Hughes et al., 1972).

The combined effects of this research point to epidemics in heroin use between 1950 and 1969. This conclusion, however, has not been universally accepted. It has been claimed that peaks on these curves are a statistical artifact due to the time clients wait to enter treatment, and the peaks which appear at the same year for successive admission cohorts are caused by a general increase in that waiting time (Richman, 1974, 1975). The waiting times are the delay from year of first heroin use to an admission to treatment. The existence of conflicting explanations reflects a mixture of information in the data about incidence and waiting time when admission data are used to estimate the distribution of users by year of first use.

Researchers often use clients who enter treatment for the first time. For these clients, the time from first use to admission is a measure of the first waiting time, and it is not mixed with waiting times that are due to repeated treatment experiences. This chapter explores how to make better use of the number of prior treatment experiences.

A MODEL FOR WAITING TIME AND INCIDENCE

For theoretical reasons, if data from an admission cohort for a particular year is graphed in relation to year of first use in order to make inferences about incidence, these data will show the effects due not only to incidence, but also to waiting time.

Confounding of the information about one of these variables will not be present if the other variable has a uniform (constant) distribution. A uniform waiting time distribution is shown in section (a) of Figure 1 as the flat horizontal line representing the same probability for waiting each number of years to enter treatment. The flat line in section (c) of Figure 1 represents uniform (constant) incidence because the same number of people begin heroin use in each year shown. Pursuant to these possibilities, it has been recognized that a peak on a year of onset curve could be due to either a peak in incidence or the mode of a waiting time distribution (Richman, 1974, 1975, 1976; and Chapter 3). These results are easily predicted by the model of incidence and waiting time presented here.

The distribution of an admission cohort by year of first use (onset) will be called an "admissions distribution." It can be shown that if incidence is constant, the admissions distribution generates a waiting time curve; and if waiting time is uniform, the admission distribution generates an incidence curve. First it will be assumed that incidence is constant. To highlight this situation, an extreme possibility will be examined.

The curve with the sharp peak in section (a) of Figure 1 represents the situation in which all clients wait five years to enter treatment. As an example, the artificial data for the curves presented in section (b) of Figure 1 show clients who entered treatment for the first time in 1975 as they are distributed over their year of first use. In this example, if every client waited five years to enter treatment, all admissions during 1975 would report 1970 as the year of first use. The percent of clients with first use in a given year (such as 1970) translates into the percent of clients who waited a particular number of years which is equal to the admission year minus the first-use year (in this case 1975 – 1970 = 5). Following this path of reasoning, it is seen that both sharp peaks in Figure 1 are located five years before admission. In fact, one can see that the waiting-time distribution in section (a) is a mirror image (an image around the vertical axis) of the curve presented in section (b). Thus, the five-year waiting time of section (a) is directly related to the curve representing distribution of admissions shown in section (b), and vice versa.

The curve in section (a) with the peak (mode) around three years represents a more realistic waiting time distribution with the time clients wait shown on the horizontal axis and the probability of a particular wait occurring on the vertical axis. In order to simplify this presentation, it will be assumed that the distribution of waiting time to enter treatment does not depend on the year of the first use (i.e., it is the same for each year of first use).

The waiting time curve in section (a) corresponds to the admissions distribution curve in section (b) with a peak or mode at 1972 (1975 − 1972 = 3 years waiting time). This mode indicates that most people in this admission cohort began heroin use in that year (remember that incidence was assumed to be constant). If this curve is reversed to make a mirror image of itself and is placed on the waiting time axis in section (a), the result is a waiting time curve with a mode (or peak) at approximately three years. This implies that most people wait about three years to enter treatment with the variation from this time represented

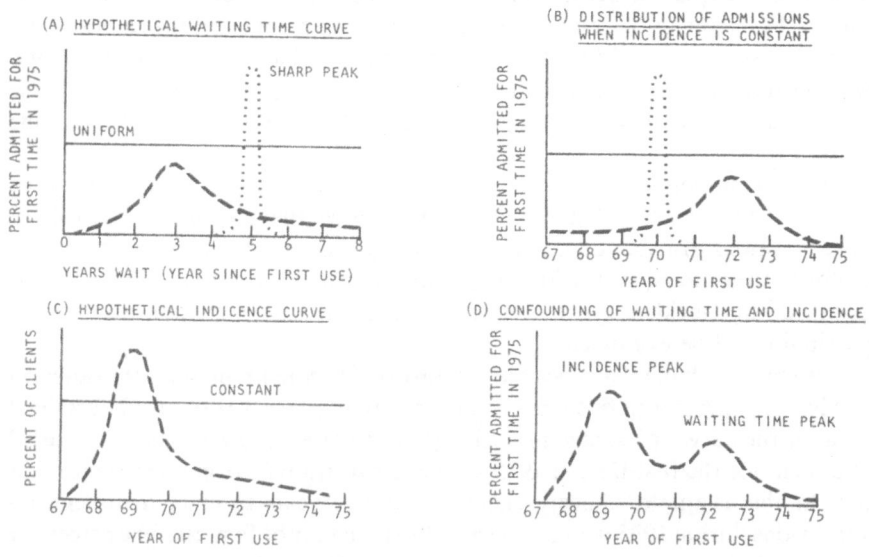

NOTE: THE CURVES REPRESENT ARTIFICIAL DATA AND ARE USED FOR ILLUSTRATIVE PURPOSES ONLY.

Fig. 1. A Model For Waiting Time and Incidence

by the sloping of the curve in both directions. The period from 1975 back to the year of onset would be the waiting time, and the percentage of clients in that year of onset would be the probability of that waiting time.

In contrast, instead of incidence being constant from year to year, let us assume that there was a large peak in incidence around 1969 as shown in Figure 1, section (c). Let us also assume that the probability of waiting different years to enter treatment is the same for each onset year, i.e., the distribution of waiting time is uniform (this would be represented by the horizontal curve in section (a), representing a constant waiting time). Under these conditions, the data from an admission cohort for 1975 showing the percent of clients in relation to their year of first heroin use measure the profile of incidence over those years. The hypothetical admissions distribution of this type becomes the one shown in section (c) of Figure 1. On this curve, a peak (or mode) is seen in 1969 with a sharp rise preceding it, and a rapid decline following it. In epidemiological terms, this pattern shows evidence of an epidemic in heroin use which peaked in 1969 and abated thereafter. Notice that section (c) illustrates both an incidence curve (hypothetical) and the same incidence curve as derived from admission when the waiting time distribution is uniform.

The examples described above show the ideal situation which would allow separate measurement of waiting time and incidence using admission data. In reality, however, different conditions exist. Evidence has been presented that incidence is not constant, and also that waiting time distributions are not uniform (Green and Dupont, 1974; Dupont and Greene, 1973; Richman, 1974; Hunt, 1974). Consequently, confounding of the information about these two variables exists. The distribution of an admission cohort according to year of first use can be derived from knowledge of the true incidence curve (number of new cases in each year) and the waiting time to enter treatment. On the other hand, if the distribution of an admission cohort according to year of first use is known, there may be an infinite number of combinations of incidence curves and waiting time distributions that will produce the observed admission cohort. Unless one finds a way to separate incidence from waiting time peaks, alternate explanations will continue to make questionable whether the 1969 peak was due to an epidemic or whether it was merely a statistical artifact caused by the waiting time peak.

A hypothetical curve based on 1975 admissions showing the mixture of information about waiting time and incidence is seen in section (d) of Figure 1. To identify the reasons for the two peaks on this curve, it is necessary to combine waiting time and incidence information from their separate sources for the same year of onset. In doing this, it will be assumed that the true incidence is shown by the curve in section (c) and that the actual waiting time distribution is that which appears in section (a) with the mode at three years. Let us consider the year of first use, 1969, which represents a waiting time of six years. Although the probability of waiting six years (from 1969 to 1975) is small, the incidence is so large in 1969 that plotting data for that year will show a peak on the curve in 1969. This gives insight into large incidence, but is misleading if related to waiting time.

The situation is reversed when the year of first use is 1972. Although the incidence was small in that year, the probability of waiting three years is relatively large and the product of the two produces a noticeable, but smaller, peak in 1972. This peak is due to more people entering treatment after a three-year wait than those waiting more or less than three years to enter treatment. The result would suggest a peak of three years for waiting time, but it may be confused with an epidemic peak.

Unlike the artificial data presented in Figure 1, real waiting time curves may not have sharp peaks. Furthermore, the peak of the waiting time curve may coincide with the peak of the incidence curve. Under these types of conditions, the distribution of one admission cohort according to year of fist use (such as Figure 1, section (d)) will not have two distinguishable peaks. For example, if one were to use admissions data from 1973, and the waiting time peak was about three years, then the waiting time peak would be around 1970, about the same year of incidence peak for the suspected 1969 epidemic. The relative sizes of the waiting time and incidence peaks, and their distance (separation) in time determine whether zero, one, or two peaks will appear in the curves. It is also conceivable that one of the peaks may appear as a small bump on the side of the major peak.

The peaks due to incidence and waiting time that are anticipated in an admissions distribution based on the preceding theoretical model may depend on the admission cohort used. For example, if the waiting time peak is about three years, it will show as a peak in 1971 with a 1974 admissions cohort and as a peak in 1973 with a 1976 admissions cohort. In fact, if only one peak is observed in an admissions distribution, the peak may be attributed to either an incidence peak or a waiting time distribution.

Let us consider the case when only one peak is found, and it is observed consistently at the same year of first use for successive admissions cohorts (such as 1974 and 1975). If the peak is attributed to waiting time, then a conclusion may be drawn that waiting time has shifted. On the other hand, if the peak year remains constant, this may be considered as evidence that a peak in incidence occurred that year. However, if two peaks appear on the graph of the admissions distribution, then it would be expected that the peak year due to incidence is at the same year for each admissions cohort, but the peak due to waiting time may occur at different years depending on the year of the admissions cohort.

METHODS

The model presented here has shown that peaks on the distribution of admissions by year of first use may be attributed to waiting time (lag) or incidence. The conceptual framework represented by the model suggests a procedure to distriminate (i.e., separate) the peaks according to effects due to waiting time or incidence. Consider plots of the distribution of admissions for various population (admission) cohorts that share some characteristics. Let those common characteristics (such as age, race and sex distribution and geographic location at time of drug abuse) be such that one expects all cohorts to have participated in an epidemic of drug abuse (if indeed one existed) around 1969. That is, the incidence curve for those cohorts would have a peak around 1969. Furthermore, let the waiting time distributions be related in some manner to the type of admission cohort. Under those conditions, the peak attributed to waiting time may not occur at the same year for all cohorts. The objective then is to compare admission distributions for cohorts that have similar incidence (same peak year) and possible different waiting time peaks year. (Lag may be different from one cohort to another.)

The data in this study is taken from the Client Oriented Data Acquisition Process (CODAP) for those clients admitted to treatment during the last half of 1974, all of 1975, and the first half of 1976. CODAP is a federal reporting requirement for all federally funded drug abuse treatment programs (Siguel and Spillane, 1975).

The population of clients is described by characteristics such as drug of abuse, type of admission, age, and admission date. The clients considered used heroin daily as primary drug of abuse and had no secondary drug problem. Clients readmitted during the period of this study were eliminated in order to avoid counting the same client twice. In addition, to eliminate atypical heroin users and possible erroneous data, clients who were younger than 12 or older than 60 were omitted. The year of first use is the year clients used heroin for the first time.

Comparisons are made across populations which differ in treatment experiences and type of admission. The two treatment experience groups consisted of those with no prior treatment and those with one or more prior treatment experiences. On the average, a much longer waiting time exists for clients who enter treatment for the nth time than for clients who enter treatment for the $(n - 1)$th time (in particular, the first time.) The waiting time distribution to enter treatment for the second to nth time is a curve reflecting the cumulative effects of separate curves for waiting time between each treatment experience. Its peak is not likely to be sharp and it must be further away from the admission year than the peak of the distribution of the waiting time to the first treatment experience. However, the incidence peak, if an epidemic has occurred, is likely to be the same for both curves.

The three admission groups are determined by the source of referral or legal status of clients admitted. They consist of three mutually exclusive and exhaustive admission groups: (a) voluntary admissions not in prison, (b) involuntary admission or TASC (Treatment Alternative to Street Crime), but not in prison, and (c) clients in prison.

RESULTS AND DISCUSSION

Figure 2 shows a pair of admission distributions by year of first use for the two treatment experience groups (no prior experience and one or more prior experiences) voluntarily admitted during 1975. Both curves have a peak around 1969 and the curve for those clients with no prior experience has a second peak at 1972. The same type of admission distributions for the other two admissions groups are displayed in Figures 3 and 4. All curves show a first peak about 1969, while the second peak in the curves depends on the type of admission and the number of treatment experiences.

In another study, extensive numerical calculations (simulations) have been used to show that a peak on onset curves can be due to waiting time alone if incidence is uniform (Richman, 1976). The model presented here easily predicts those results and extends the investigation beyond it (i.e., these results are a special case of the general model). The curves for those clients who have no prior

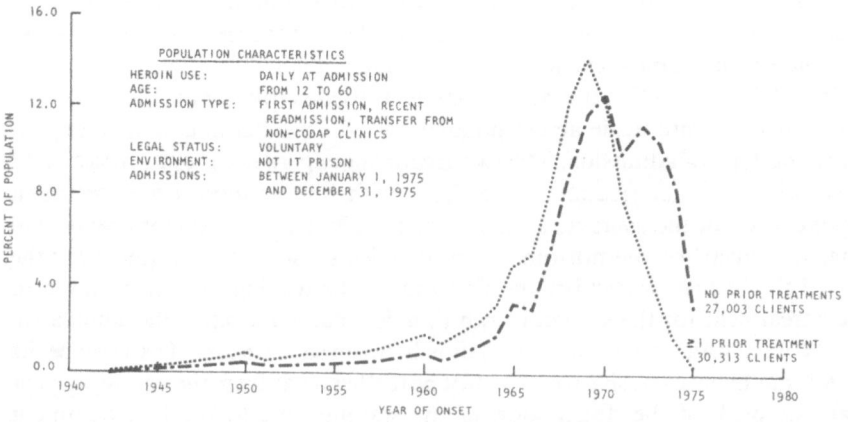

Fig. 2. Distribution of number of prior treatment experiences in relation to the year of first use

treatment experience measure the first waiting time to admission as well as incidence. If incidence were constant, there would be one peak for waiting time, but the curves in this study show two peaks. There can be little doubt that the consistent peaks are due to incidence. As a result, it seems that the controversy concerning a peak in incidence about 1969 is now resolved.

The absence of a second peak on the curve for clients with one or more prior treatment experiences is seen to be the result of larger mean waiting times for this group and a flatter distribution of waiting times which causes the peak to be subsumed within the incidence peak.

The existence of a constant peak about 1969 due to incidence and the second peak on the no prior experience curve due to waiting time found in Figure 2 was further substantiated by repeating the two curves for two additional admission groups. Figure 3 shows the same two types of curves for those who are involuntary admissions or in TASC, but not in prison, for all of 1975. Again, both curves have a peak about 1969. In this case, the onset curve for no prior treatment experience shows two peaks, one at 1972 and the other at 1974. In addition, the curve representing the group with one or more prior experiences also has a second peak at 1974.

Figure 4 displays the pair of onset curves for the two treatment groups treated in the prison environment during 1975. Again, both curves have peaks at about 1969 while the curve for no prior treatment experience has a distinct second peak at 1972.

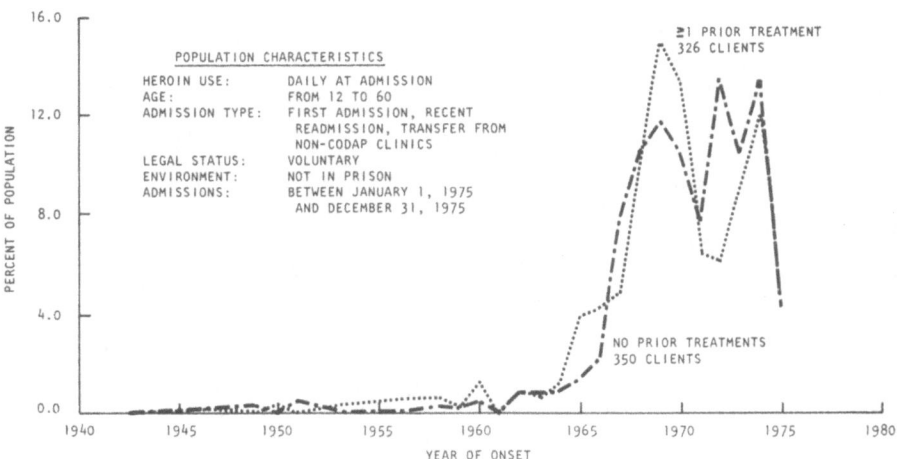

Fig. 3. Distribution of number of prior treatment experiences in relation to the year of first use

There are several interesting characteristics in the data. The second peak attributed to waiting time varies in size and location according to the type of admission (as expected). The curves for involuntary admissions have a new peak at around 1974, which does not appear in any of the other population groups. It should be noted that the same peak appears in the curves for clients with no prior treatment experiences as well as clients with prior treatment experiences. This result will occur if the waiting-time distributions for the nth treatment experience are multimodal precisely in a fashion that would produce another peak in 1974. However, this is highly unlikely because the waiting-time distributions depend on the number of prior treatment experiences and should not have peaks at the same year.

A more tenable explantion is that a substantial increase in incidence during 1974 (as compared with 1973) accounts for the 1974 peak. This peak is evident in the involuntary curves and not in the voluntary or prison environment curves because the probability of an involuntary admission one year after first use is much larger, on the average, than the corresponding probability for voluntary admissions or those in prison (since it takes a long time to be processed by the judicial system). An increase in incidence in 1974 would not be reflected in incidence curves for voluntary admissions or clients in prison for at least one more year because since the probability of waiting one year to enter treatment is quite small, even a large incidence in 1974 would still produce a small number of admissions in 1975. The 1972 peak in the involuntary admissions with no prior

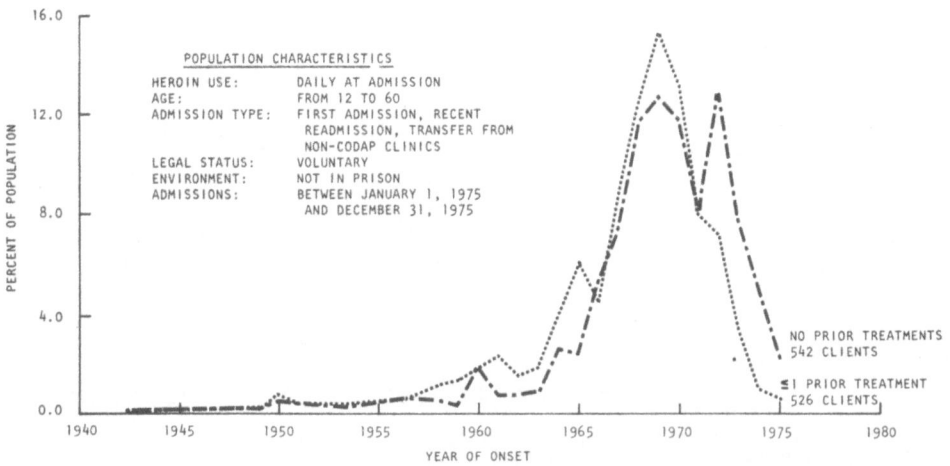

Fig. 4. Distribution of number of prior treatment experiences in relation to the year of first use

treatment is attributable to the average waiting time to enter treatment for the first time.

It has been argued that involuntary admissions reflect the emphasis of the judicial process on referring clients for treatment and are therefore not valid indicators of incidence. However, judges are not likely to use the year clients began to use drugs as a basis to decide whether or not to refer a client for treatment. An increase in incidence for 1974, therefore, will not be due to an increase in the number of referrals. An increase in the number of referrals would about equally affect all years of first use in the range 1970-1975 and could not produce the large 1974 peak shown by the data. The view that the increase in 1974 reflects an increase in incidence is supported by preliminary tabulations on heroin indicators prepared by the National Institute on Drug Abuse (1976).

After the criticisms of employing distributions of admission cohorts in relation to year of first heroin use have been considered, it can still be seen that such distributions can be used to identify trends in incidence. Of course, care must be taken to control the confounding influence of waiting time. When this is done, admission distributions become a viable method for detecting changes in incidence. The data presented here suggest that there was an epidemic about 1969, followed by a decrease in incidence until 1973, and an increase again in 1974.

REFERENCES

De Alarcon, R., "The spread of heroin abuse in a community," *U.N. Bulletin on Narcotics,* 21 (1969), 17-22.

Dupont, R.L. and Greene, M.H., "The dynamics of a heroin addiction epidemic," *Science,* 181 (1973), 716-722.

Greene, M.H. and Dupont, R.L., Heroin addiction trends," *Amer. J. Psychiatry,* 131 (1974), 545-550.

Greene, M.H., Luke, J.L., and Dupont, K.L., "Opiate overdose deaths in the District of Columbia: Heroin-related fatalities," *Med. Ann. of the District of Columbia,* 43, (1974), 175-181.

Huber, D.H., Stivers, R.R., and Howard, L.B., "Heroin overdose deaths in Atlanta: An epidemic," *JAMA,* 228 (1974), 319-322.

Hughes, P.H., Barker, N.W., Crawford, G.A., and Jaffe, J.H., "The natural-history of a heroin epidemic," *Am. J. Public Health,* 62 (1972), 955-1001.

Hughes, P.H. and Crawford, G.A., "A contagious disease model for researching and intervening in heroin epidemics," *Arch. Gen. Psychiatry,* 27 (1972), 149-155.

Hunt, L.G., "Recent spread of heroin in the United States," *Am. J. Public Health Supplement,* 64 (1974), 16-23.

Ipsen, J., Cuskey, W.R., and Premkumar, T., "Deaths from medicaments in relation to epidemic drug addiction," *Internat. J. Epidemiology* 2 (1973), 329-337.

Levengood, R., Lowinger, P., and Schoof, K., "Heroin addiction in the suburbs: An epidemiological study," *Am. J. Public Health,* 63 (1973), 209-214.

Minichiello, L. and Retka, R., "Trends in intravenous drug abuse as reflected in national hepatitis reporting," *Am. J. Public Health,* 66 (1976).

National Institute on Drug Abuse, *Heroin Indicators Trend Report, July 1976,* DHEW Publication N, (ADM) 76-378, 1976.

Newmeyer, J.A., "Further Notes on the Heroin Epidemic in San Francisco Bay Area," paper presented to the North American Congress on Alcohol and Drug Problems, San Francisco, 1974.

Richman, A., "Epidemiological Assessment of Changes in the Onset of Narcotic Addiction," *Proceedings of the 36th Annual Meeting of the Committee on Problems of Drug Dependence,* Mexico City, 1974.

Richman, A., "Heroin Addict Forecasting—Statistical Fallacies and Disputed Facts," *Proceeding of the Social Statistics Section of the American Statistical Association, 1975.*

Richman, A., "Pseudo Epidemics," paper presented at American Public Health Association Meeting, Miami, 1976.

Siguel, E.N. and Spillane, W.H., "The Client Oriented Data Acquisition Process (CODAP)," National Institute on Drug Abuse, Rockville, Md., 1975.

CHAPTER 3

The Retail Price of Heroin: Estimation and Applications

GEORGE F. BROWN, JR.
LESTER P. SILVERMAN

This article develops estimates of the retail price of heroin in a number of U.S. cities and applies them to problems associated with the use of illicit narcots. Our retail price estimates, based on purchases of heroin by narcotics enforcement agents, show considerable fluctuation over time, a fact not reported systematically before. The estimated price series provide insight into the structure of the heroin market and the relationship between heroin availability and crime.

The planning and evaluation of public policy toward drug abuse has, in the past, been hampered by a lack of meaningful statistics. Such variables as the numbers of addicts, the production, consumption, and availability of illicit drugs, and the numbers of drug-related deaths or illnesses are difficult to define, much less observe and measure. Empirical studies based on these and other variables have therefore suffered.

One measure of the relative availability of illicit narcotics on which some data have been collected is price. While we would prefer, ideally, to estimate the demand and supply curves generating equilibrium prices, prices can be interpreted as a measure of relative availability. Policy issues, such as the effect of law enforcement activities on availability of drugs and the effect of changes in market conditions on the drug user, can thus be addressed with price data.

To date, the only systematic information on the prices of illicit drugs was provided in monthly reports by field agents of the Bureau of Narcotics and Dangerous Drugs (BNDD) on their Form 199, "The Availability and Prices of Illicit Drugs." These data have two crucial deficiencies for analytical purposes. First, only wide ranges of price, purity, and quantity are reported. Second, the ranges do not change much over time. Price may fluctuate markedly across time, while remaining within the ranges reported. For example, in New York City the same ranges on price, purity, and quantity were quoted from June 1970 through November 1971; the price per gram of heroin during this period could have varied between $8.80 and $233 and still have fallen within the quoted ranges. These deficiencies are found in data reported for other cities and other periods as well.

Using an alternative data source, reports of purchases of illicit drugs by narcotics enforcement officers, we have estimated the relationship between the price per gram of heroin paid by the purchaser and the quantity and purity of the purchase and the month in which it took place. These estimated relationships are used to infer the price per gram which prevailed in that city for each month for a "standardized" retail purchase.

The methodology for constructing the price series is presented, as are price series for three cities—New York, Detroit and Los Angeles. The resulting analysis provides insights into the structure of the heroin distribution system and the relationship between market conditions and crime. These subjects are discussed in turn.

ESTIMATION OF PRICE SERIES

Model of the Heroin Market

Heroin entering the U.S. passes through many hands before reaching our cities' streets. Previous studies (Preble and Casey, 1969; Moore, 1972a) have estimated that six distinct middlemen insulate the heroin importer and extract profits from the distribution of successively smaller and more diluted quantities of the narcotic.

The total quantity of heroin supplied in a given city at a specific time (H_S) is considered a function of the retail price of heroin $(P/Q)^*$, the average quantity (Q) and potency (S) of a transaction, the activities of law enforcement (L) agencies, and the availability of the narcotic to the wholesalers (V). The rationale for inclusion of quantity and potency in the supply equation is discussed shortly. The total quantity demanded (H_D) is a function of the retail

price, the number of addicts (N), and the relative attractiveness of heroin (A).
With the market clearing equilibrium condition $H_S = H_D = H$, we have

$$H = f_1[(P/Q)^*, Q, S, L, V],$$
$$H = f_2[(P/Q)^*, N, A].$$

The reduced-form equations for this system are:

$$P^*/Q = g_1(Q, S, L, V, N, A),$$
$$H = g_2(Q, S, L, V, N, A).$$

We have no observations on the total quantity of heroin transacted in the illicit market, and thus are not able to estimate the second equation. The price equation also contains variables for which measures are not available. We assume that the level of law enforcement, availability of imported heroin, number of addicts, and degree of addiction are all relatively constant over the period of a month. This is especially crucial with regard to the relative attractiveness of heroin (V) which is affected by the price of heroin, the price of substitute drugs, and the availability of treatment programs. Since data do not exist to estimate this implied simultaneous-equations model, we must assume that V is predetermined in the reduced-form equation for price.

Thus, while we cannot separate the effects of the various supply and demand factors, we can estimate the monthly variation in prices, for a given quantity and potency, due to the total of these forces. Future work will attempt to separate the relative influence of these several factors on the availability of retail heroin, as reflected in its price.

Data

The price series we have estimated are based on reports of tests performed by BNDD laboratories on heroin and other drugs purchased by federal, state, and local narcotics agents from July 1970 through June 1972. Each report shows the date, place, and cost of each purchase, as well as a description of the drug as stated by the seller. The laboratories, in addition, report the actual composition of the drug purchased, the quantity (usually in grams), and the potency (in percentage of purity). Data were available for 41 cities, but reasonably complete series for the two-year period could only be estimated for nine major cities. Series for New York, Detroit, and Los Angeles are presented here; series for the other major cities are found in Brown and Silverman (1973).

Difficulties in constructing the price series arose because these data were collected as a side result of enforcement efforts rather than from a planned

survey. The main methodological problem resulted from the fact that purchases
were made at many levels of quantity and purity, reflecting the operations of
enforcement agents at various levels of the heroin market.

Some of the agents' purchases were made at the retail or street level where
quantities are small and potencies are low; others were made far up the
distribution chain. The shortage of obviously retail purchases in each month
leads us to follow a procedure in which all the purchases in a month are used to
estimate a retail price for a unit of standard quantity and purity.

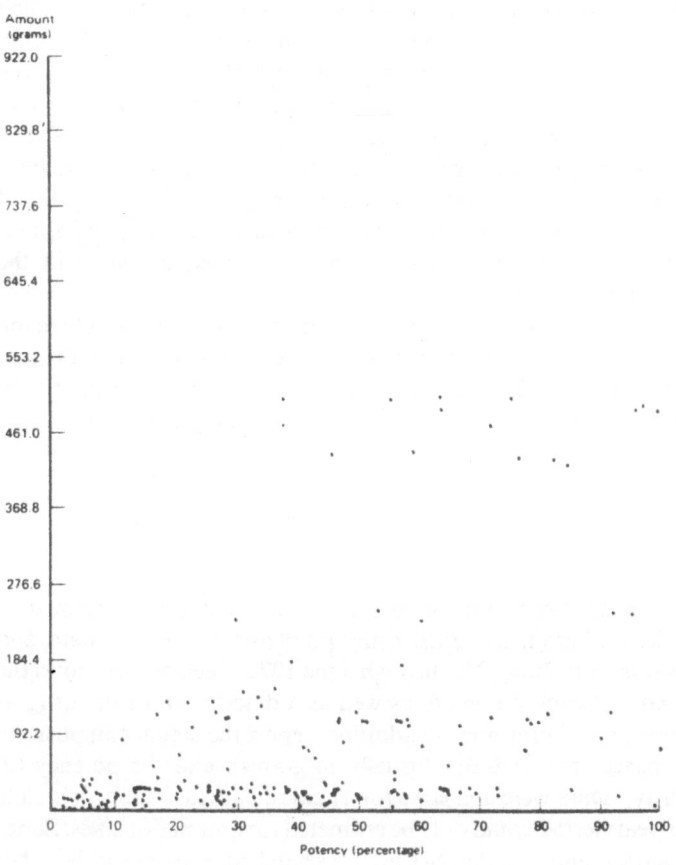

Fig. 1. Plot of Quantity and Potency of Heroin Buys in New York City/Manhattan

Figure 1 shows a scatter plot of the quantities and purities of all 217 purchases made in the Manhattan borough of New York City. Purchases were made over a broad range of quantity and purity, reflecting the fact that enforcement agents were operating at all wholesale and retail levels of the heroin market. Enforcement-related buys also varied from month to month. In New York, the number of buys varied from zero (in one month early in the two-year period under study) to as many as 29 in June 1971. Such variation was also found in the number of purchases and in the quantity and potency at which purchases were made in the other cities covered by our data.

Before discussing the methodology employed to use these data for estimating price, it is necessary to address the question of whether the BNDD purchase data are useful at all. Are purchases made by enforcement agents, for ultimate use in enforcement, reflective of prices prevailing in the actual addict market?

The representativeness of the buys made by enforcement agents depends on their coverage of local market; the extent of their coverage is unknown. Enforcement agents may be buying from relatively new suppliers to minimize their risk, or they may be relatively well entrenched in the local market and able to purchase at lower prices. Whatever the bias inherent in these buys, we presume it is consistent across the period of our data, leading to correct estimates of relative fluctuations, although absolute levels may be incorrect.

One indicator of the performance of the agents who make the buys is the frequency of "ripoffs," i.e., unknowing purchases of substances that contain no heroin. In New York City, Chicago, Detroit, and Los Angeles, four of the cities for which we have the most data, the percentages of buys that turned out to be "ripoffs" are 2.7, 0.0, 6.8, and 2.0, respectively. These figures appear to be reasonable for transactions in this market and provide some indication of the effectiveness of these agents. Enforcement agents at various levels have suggested that because of the agents' knowledge about and continuing presence in the heroin market, their purchases are reflective of actual market conditions.

We later present evidence that these price estimates are in general consistent with previously published point estimates and with *a priori* expectations relating to such incidents as the East Coast dock strike.

Methodology

Deletion of Outliers

A test for consistency in the buy data is made by estimating the parameters of

$$P_i = \beta_0 Q_i^{\beta_1} S_i^{\beta_2} T_i^{\beta_3} v_i \qquad (1)$$

where:

> P_i = price paid for ith buy (dollars),
> Q_i = quantity of ith buy (grams),
> S_i = purity of ith buy (percent),
> T_i = month of purchase.

Equation (1) is estimated, for each city, in multiplicative form (and hence linear in the logs of the variables) because of the interaction of quantity and potency in determining price. Because of the nature of the heroin distribution system, the effect of an increase in potency, for example, on price should depend on the quantity bought. The multiplicative functional form is thus superior from a theoretical (and empirical) view. The log of the error term v_i is assumed to have zero mean and finite variance.

The explanatory power of this model is over 90 percent for 24 of the cities, and under 80 percent for only four. Individual residuals that exceeded three times their estimated standard error were examined carefully. In each case, the price paid was clearly out of line with the quantity and purity of the purchase. For example, according to one of the three New York/Manhattan outliers, the agent purchased 0.3 grams of 23.4 percent heroin for $1,000, a price of $14,245 per pure gram. (The average price per gram (P/SQ) for Manhattan is $231.) In our opinion, a coding or keypunch error is the cause of this outlier and most others. The number of observations deleted was actually quite small (only one each in Boston, Houston, Los Angeles and Miami; two each in Baltimore and Detroit; and three each in Chicago, New York and New Orleans). Their effect on the results, however, is significant.

Estimation of Standardized Price

Table 1 shows time series of the price per gram and price per pure gram of heroin in New York City. We obtain these series by simply averaging all purchases for a given month after deleting purchases involving ripoffs and outliers (as just discussed). Table 1 also shows the number of observations (purchases) available in the preparation of each month's price statistics. Note that considerably more observations are available later in the reporting period, a fact generally true for all cities, probably because of problems associated with setting up the computerized data system, but potentially reflecting changes in enforcement policy. The price-per-gram series shows considerably more stability than does the price-per-pure-gram series, fluctuating only within the range of about $20-50.

One problem with both of these series is that they are based on data from

**Table 1. Unadjusted Number of Buys and Price Series
for New York City/Manhattan**

Month/year	Number of observations	Unadjusted Price/gram (P/Q)	Unadjusted Price/pure gram (P/SQ)
7/70	4	30.10	52.83
8/70	2	20.77	23.12
9/70	4	–	–
10/70	1	19.54	21.52
11/70	1	20.64	20.64
12/70	2	27.50	52.55
1/71	1	38.56	91.38
2/71	2	42.86	84.54
3.71	2	30.91	73.64
4/71	5	40.77	97.37
5/71	9	38.96	175.00
6/71	29	42.22	185.27
7/71	5	39.47	221.32
8/71	14	43.47	104.57
9/71	12	50.85	113.75
10/71	19	49.52	151.96
11/71	11	40.64	164.98
12/71	3	39.99	640.76
1/72	14	50.95	211.04
2/72	19	40.43	153.61
3/72	16	41.96	159.03
4/72	19	37.83	793.81
5/72	19	36.41	312.16
6/72	8	44.87	240.01

purchases at different levels of the distribution system. The nature of enforcement activities may have led to purchases transacted at the street level in one month, and, in another month, further up the distribution system.

Because of both the changing nature of the risk involved and the value added to the product by the activities of middle men, there is reason to believe that the price at which a gram of heroin can be bought is affected by the quantity and purity of the purchase made. A supplier may be willing to charge less per gram when selling a larger quantity of heroin, since the number of transactions—and, presumably, the risk—are lower.

A higher purity level of the substance being purchased is associated with a higher price per gram, but presumably a lower price per pure gram, since the value normally added by dilution and distribution is absent. Thus, the series in Table 1 is tainted by the nature of the enforcement activity, as reflected in

Table 2. Estimated Coefficients and R^2 of Price/Gram Equation*
(t-values in parentheses)

City	β_0	β_1	β_2	β_3	R^2	Number
Albuquerque	8.17	−0.22	0.14	−1.53	.579	41
		(−6.47)	(1.44)	(−4.60)		
Atlanta	4.39	−0.11	0.16	−0.21	.201	47
		(−2.84)	(2.09)	(−0.62)		
Baltimore	4.06	−0.28	0.12	−0.03	.518	59
		(−7.19)	(1.54)	(−0.21)		
Boston	3.09	−0.16	0.09	0.36	.372	60
		(−3.82)	(0.89)	(3.76)		
Boulder	−27.10	0.14	2.00	9.42	.842	5
		(0.53)	(0.91)	(0.29)		
Buffalo	9.97	−0.97	0.05	−2.30	.929	45
		(−22.97)	(0.51)	(−12.70)		
Chicago	3.58	−0.22	0.29	0.02	.412	115
		(−8.11)	(5.72)	(0.25)		
Cleveland	1.95	−0.23	−0.04	0.83	.611	27
		(−4.47)	(−0.52)	(2.41)		
Dallas	3.72	−0.29	0.14	0.17	.790	22
		(−6.99)	(0.68)	(0.66)		
Denver	6.84	−0.41	−0.09	−0.84	.839	46
		(−10.86)	(−1.14)	(−3.33)		
Detroit	2.98	−0.17	0.25	0.21	.439	123
		(−8.06)	(6.11)	(3.06)		
Hartford	2.91	−0.16	0.07	0.46	.835	23
		(−4.86)	(0.68)	(6.09)		
Honolulu	6.27	−0.80	−0.04	−0.08	.999	5
		(−12.79)	(−7.74)	(−12.75)		
Houston	4.78	−0.41	0.09	−0.13	.843	61
		(−14.49)	(0.98)	(−1.59)		
Indianapolis	7.81	−0.25	−0.26	−0.87	.711	13
		(−3.51)	(−1.04)	(−0.74)		
Jacksonville	4.59	−0.31	−0.14	0.10	.816	10
		(−4.77)	(−1.07)	(0.69)		
Kansas City	4.92	−0.32	0.02	−0.14	.768	38
		(−8.48)	(0.30)	(−1.13)		
Los Angeles	3.72	−0.15	−0.05	0.04	.352	97
		(−6.05)	(−1.08)	(0.83)		
Memphis	1.49	−0.42	0.18	0.91	.688	36
		(−7.11)	(2.26)	(1.15)		
Miami	4.00	−0.22	0.25	−0.07	.478	79
		(−8.04)	(3.58)	(−0.41)		
Milwaukee	5.20	−0.46	0.25	−0.17	.819	8
		(−2.64)	(0.67)	(−0.19)		

Table 2. Continued)

City	β_0	β_1	β_2	β_3	R^2	Number
Minneapolis	−11.80	1.56 (5.10)	4.10 (7.95)	0.81 (3.31)	.974	7
New York/New Jersey	5.69	−0.29 (−4.18)	0.32 (3.20)	−0.69 (−0.28)	.598	18
New York/Long Island	3.77	−0.34 (−2.34)	0.46 (1.38)	−0.22 (−0.51)	.451	11
New York/Bronx	2.86	−0.22 (−3.16)	0.35 (3.58)	0.14 (1.02)	.379	30
New York/Brooklyn	3.38	−0.15 (−4.90)	0.18 (2.52)	0.07 (1.13)	.375	49
New York/Manhattan	2.81	−0.17 (−8.36)	0.30 (9.39)	0.14 (2.78)	.345	217
Nashville	3.62	0.04 (0.44)	0.19 (1.36)	0.02 (0.02)	.063	35
New Orleans	2.00	−0.27 (−13.68)	0.39 (9.44)	0.52 (4.71)	.826	104
Philadelphia	3.64	−0.40 (−4.75)	0.42 (3.73)	0.43 (0.19)	.730	24
Phoenix	3.95	−0.29 (−13.12)	0.09 (1.25)	0.05 (0.16)	.881	34
Pittsburgh	3.12	0.01 (0.06)	0.12 (0.73)	0.23 (0.87)	.134	13
Portland	3.01	−0.23 (−5.81)	0.18 (2.69)	0.28 (1.93)	.883	16
San Antonio	4.54	−0.20 (−5.49)	−0.23 (−1.29)	0.04 (0.36)	.712	17
San Francisco area	6.36	−0.04 (−0.32)	0.40 (4.45)	−1.31 (−4.33)	.969	6
San Francisco	4.75	−0.22 (−4.62)	−0.06 (−0.87)	−0.20 (−1.73)	.564	29
Seattle	2.35	−0.28 (−6.65)	0.37 (4.28)	0.48 (4.01)	.615	45
St. Louis	3.01	−0.27 (−5.35)	−0.04 (−0.29)	0.52 (1.85)	.570	54
Tampa	−46.42	−0.34 (−1.11)	0.49 (2.07)	16.21 (1.20)	.397	14
Tucson	4.90	−0.43 (−16.03)	0.39 (5.15)	−0.34 (−1.35)	.991	9
Washington, D.C.	2.31	−0.21 (−5.49)	0.52 (11.21)	0.19 (1.91)	.779	56

*Log $P/Q = \beta_0 + \beta_1$ Log q + β_2 Log S + β_3 Log T

the different quantities and purities associated with the purchases, and is not reflective of standard retail purchases.

We thus consider the structural relation

$$(P/Q)_i = \beta_0 Q_i^{\beta_1} S_i^{\beta_2} T_i^{\beta_3} u_i, \tag{2}$$

where all symbols are as previously defined. The price per gram of each purchase is a function of the quantity and purity of the buy (as suggested by the model of the distribution system), of the month of purchase, and of other, unobserved factors such as law enforcement, supply conditions, number of addicts, degree of addiction, which are incorporated in the disturbance term u_i. Estimation of (6) for each city yields values for the parameters $\beta_0, \beta_1, \beta_2, \beta_3$, and, in addition, estimates of u_i, for each buy.

$$(P/Q)_i = \hat{\beta}_0 Q_i^{\hat{\beta}_1} S_i^{\hat{\beta}_2} T_i^{\hat{\beta}_3} \hat{u}_i. \tag{3}$$

Assuming that the "retail" sale at a quantity of Q^* grams and purity S^* percent occurs in the same month, we can predict the price per gram, $(P/Q)^*$, at which this "standardized" retail buy would have taken place by

$$(P/Q)^*_i = \hat{\beta}_0 (Q^*)^{\hat{\beta}_1} (S^*)^{\hat{\beta}_2} (T_i)^{\hat{\beta}_3} \hat{u}_i. \tag{4}$$

Equation (2.4) can be rewritten, with the use of (3), as follows:

$$(P/Q)^*_i = (P/Q)_i (Q^*/Q_i)^{\beta_1} (S^*/S_i)^{\beta_2} \tag{5}$$

Equation (5), with the parameters β_1 and β_2 estimated from (2), shows the estimated retail price the heroin in this purchase would have attracted at the standardized retail level.

Table 2 shows the parameters estimated for (2) for each of the 41 cities. Were it not for the deletion of outliers, the results of Table 2 would be directly recoverable from the estimated coefficients of (1)—except for the t-value of the (log) Q variable.

Price Series for Selected Cities

The results of Table 2 allow computation of a standardized price per gram $(P/Q)^*$ from (5) for each buy made in each city. We obtain monthly estimates by averaging these hypothetical buys for a given month. An implicit assumption here is that purchases made at the wholesale level would have been transacted at the retail level in the same month.

Figure 2 shows our estimates of the price per gram that prevailed in New York City in each month for a purchase made in a quantity of two grams and at a potency of ten percent (the units we have chosen as a standard); estimates of the standardized price per gram—$(P/Q)^*$—are shown in tabular and graphical form. For purposes of comparison, the price-per-gram and price-

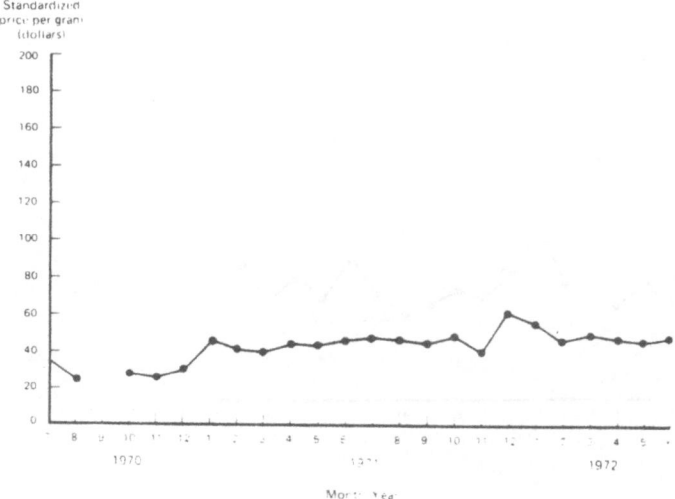

Month year	Number of observations	Unadjusted price per gram	Unadjusted price per pure gram	Adjusted price per gram
7 70	4	30 10	52 83	34 39
8 70	2	20 77	23 12	24 45
9 70	0			
10 70	1	19 54	21 52	27 97
11 70	1	20 64	20 64	25 78
12 70	2	. 27 50	52 55	29 71
1 71	1	38 56	91 38	45 77
2 71	2	42 86	84 54	41 20
3 71	2	30 91	73 64	40 14
4 71	5	40 77	97 37	44 85
5 71	9	38 96	175 00	43 40
6 71	29	42 22	185 27	46 17
7 71	5	39 47	221 32	48 00
8 71	14	43 47	104 57	47 01
9 71	12	50 85	113 75	44 70
10 71	19	49 52	151 96	49 96
11 71	11	40 64	164 98	39 79
12 71	3	39 99	640 76	61 93
1 72	14	50 95	211 04	55 95
2 72	19	40 43	153 61	46 36
3 72	16	41 96	159 03	50 08
4 72	19	37 83	793 81	47 56
5 72	19	36 41	312 16	45 76
6 72	8	44 87	240 01	48 26

Fig. 2. Adjusted Price Series for New York City/Manhattan

per-pure-gram series obtained by a simple averaging of the BNDD purchase data is replicated from Table 2.

Though the standardized and naive price-per-gram series are quite similar (their correlation is 0.83), there are differences between them, the result of enforcement activities at different levels reflected in the varying quantity and potency levels of the purchases made from month to month.

Month/ year	Number of observations	Unadjusted price per gram	Unadjusted price per pure gram	Adjusted price per gram
7/70	0		..	
8/70	4	31.86	66 37	30 53
9/70	6	40.69	70 29	46 09
10/70	2	55 21	159 36	57 93
11/70	2	91.25	135 42	45 94
12/70	1	340 91	722 27	159 56
1/71	1	54.95	250 89	51 56
2/71	4	62.94	552 99	62 25
3/71	2	39 21	198 54	50 21
4/71	0			
5/71	1	73.05	113 25	62 47
6/71	2	100.60	674 33	93 50
7/71	2	36.21	436 82	67 85
8/71	6	42 54	408 12	53 99
9/71	5	50 82	259 21	58 27
10/71	7	49 76	198 10	51 38
11/71	5	33 45	197 05	44 68
12/71	11	54 27	3400 27	56 05
1 72	2	59.32	2036 32	76 18
2 72	11	45 36	456 59	53 14
3 72	15	63 25	479 95	66 15
4/72	11	37 14	500 74	52 40
5 72	10	48 34	857 09	71 57
6 72	12	103 87	961 18	80 92

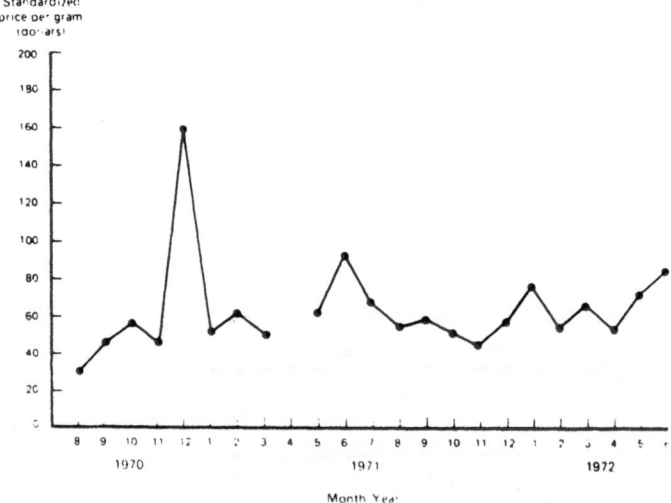

Fig. 3. Adjusted Price Series for Detroit

The New York City series (Figure 2) had only one month without observations, but only one month out of the first nine had more than two observations. From June 1971 through June 1972, the New York series is based on an average of 14 observations per month.

The standardized price series is shown in tabular and graphical form for Detroit and Los Angeles in Figures 3 and 4, respectively; also shown are the

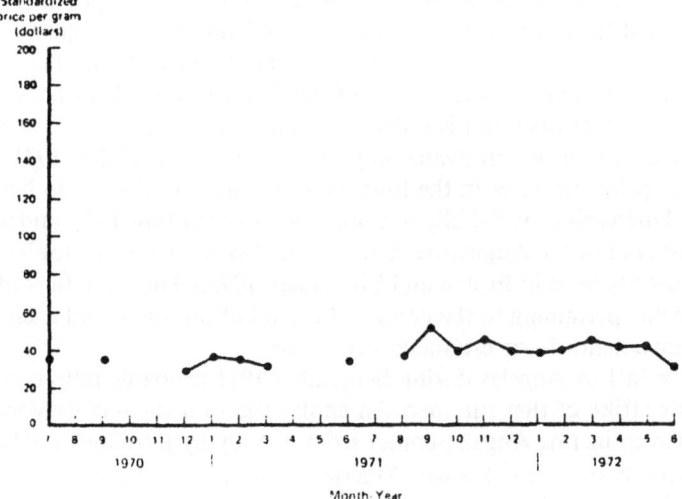

Month/ year	Number of observations	Unadjusted price per gram	Unadjusted price per pure gram	Adjusted price per gram
7/70	8	23.83	146.92	38.43
8/70	0	--	--	--
9/70	3	19.47	61.94	35.08
10/70	0	-	-	
11/70	0	-	--	
12/70	3	18.77	89.01	28.47
1/71	3	21.84	87.92	35.85
2/71	1	23.70	145.38	34.64
3/71	4	21.81	77.01	30.74
4/71	0	-		--
5/71	0	-	-	
6/71	1	21.94	74.14	33.86
7/71	0	-	-	-
8/71	2	24.12	781.12	35.21
9/71	4	38.67	568.75	50.83
10/71	3	27.32	1166.58	38.40
11/71	8	29.07	298.02	45.13
12/71	4	28.86	326.46	38.66
1/72	4	25.55	210.37	38.41
2/72	6	25.89	148.43	39.37
3/72	4	30.12	234.65	44.33
4/72	11	31.72	374.41	41.02
5/72	20	37.73	409.85	40.52
6/72	10	25.51	206.62	29.72

Fig. 4. Adjusted Price Series for Los Angeles

number of purchases in the month and, for purposes of comparison, the simple average price per gram and price per pure gram obtained from the raw data. The Detroit series has only two months for which no observations are present; Los Angeles has several in the first year of the data. For both cities, the number of observations in each month fluctuates considerably and is higher toward the end of the reporting period. Series for several other cities are presented in Brown and Silverman (1973).

The price series presented in Figures 2, 3 and 4 show that the price per gram for heroin fluctuates with differences in timing and magnitude across the cities. The series estimated for New York and Los Angeles are somewhat more stable and at a lower level of price than the series for Detroit. Upward trends in the price per gram are suggested by the series for New York and Detroit, but not for Los Angeles.

It is difficult to construct external checks on the estimated series because of the lack of independent data. One source of qualitative information (which certainly is not independent of our data base) is the monthly BNDD 199 reports in which field agents occasionally comment on market conditions. (These narratives comment on packaging as well as conditions in all drug markets, e.g., heroin, cocaine, LSD.)

The reports for New York assert that heroin was in short supply in December 1970 and January 1971 but became available again in March. These conditions are reflected in Figure 2, showing price rising to a peak of $45.77 per gram (for a purchase of two grams at 10 percent purity) in January 1971 and decreasing to $40.14 in March 1971, a relative low point. The narrative asserts that the price level remained constant from April to September 1971, a period in which our price series shows great stability. A shortage of wholesale heroin, reportedly a consequence of the East Coast dock strike, was felt in October and December and is reflected in high retail prices.

A reported decrease in heroin availability in Detroit in November 1971 is reflected in large price increases in the following two months. Agents in New Orleans reported increasing availability of wholesale heroin in June 1971, and we observe a decrease in price in August-November of that year. (The series for New Orleans, not shown here, is in Brown and Silverman, 1973.) These are the only narrative comments pertaining to the cities and period of our data, and each is reflected in a movement of our estimated price series.

The peak price in Los Angeles during September 1971 probably reflects the West Coast dock strike of that summer. An explanation for the relatively low price of retail heroin in Los Angeles comes from a study by Redlinger (1970), who declares that retail sales to Mexican-Americans take place at a relatively low price because of lower risks associated with dealing with friends and compatriots. The fact that large quantities of heroin enter the U.S. from Mexico [Committee on Government Operations (1965, p. 61)] also helps explain the lower average street prices of Los Angeles. (The same explanation applies to Houston, where BNDD estimates the lowest street prices of the major cities.)

Comparison of our series for seven cities with BNDD point estimates for December 1970 (taken from Wald and Hutt, 1972) reveal that our estimates are within the established range.

STRUCTURE OF THE HEROIN MARKET

The research conducted in constructing the price series presented in Section 2 and the price series themselves provide a basis for analysis of the structure of the heroin market. A number of these implications are discussed in this section.

Quantity and Purity Effects on Price

Various reasons were suggested for a relationship between the price per gram and the price per pure gram of heroin, on the one hand, and, on the other, the quantity and purity of the heroin purchased. The price data can be used to test these anecdotal accounts of the behavior of this market.

Because of the illicit nature of the heroin market, one might expect the risk associated with a transaction to have a bearing on the price. The risk borne by the supplier is presumably associated positively with the number of transactions he must make. (This hypothesis is discussed by Rottenberg, 1968; and Moore, 1972.) Purchases in large quantities would reduce the number of risky transactions in which the distributor would be involved. The unit price at which the supplier sells the heroin should, then, be a decreasing function of the size of the transaction. (Risk is not the only factor here; quantity discounts exist for licit goods as well.)

This hypothesis is strongly confirmed by Tabulation A, which summarizes the sign and significance of the coefficient of the quantity variable in the price per gram regressions of Table 2. For 37 of the 41 cities in our data, price per gram is a decreasing function of the number of grams of heroin bought; the t statistic is greater than two for 35 of these 37 cities. For the nine cities for which we had the most complete data, the coefficient of the quantity variable is negative and has a t statistic greater than two for each of the estimated equations. This strongly supports the presence of quantity discounts in the heroin market as a method of reducing risk, or otherwise increasing the utility of the seller.

The effect of the potency of the purchase on the price per gram and on the price per pure gram is also of interest. Clearly, the higher the percentage of heroin in the substance bought, the higher the price per gram one would expect to pay. Thus, we hypothesize a positive relationship between the price per *gram* and the potency level.

A. Sign and Significance of Quantity and Potency In Price Per Gram Regression* For All Cities

t-value	Negative	Positive
	Quantity (log Q)	
2.00 or more	35	1
less than 2.00	2	3
	Potency (log S)	
2.00 or more	1	18
less than 2.00	8	14

*$\text{Log}\,(P/Q) = \beta_0 + \beta_1 \text{Log}\,Q + \beta_2 \text{Log}\,S + \beta_3 \text{Log}\,T.$

On the other hand, one of the economic services provided by distributors in the heroin market is dilution of the drug to a level at which an addict may use it. Another economic service, distribution of the drug itself, is typically accompanied by dilution to lower levels of potency to compensate the seller for increased risks as the drug approaches the street (see Redlinger, 1970). Thus, the price per pure gram presumably increases as the narcotic flows through the distribution system, reaching a maximum at the street level. This implies that the price per *pure gram* is negatively related to the level of potency at which the drug is purchased.

Evidence from the estimated equations strongly supports these hypotheses, as demonstrated in Tabulations A and B. For 32 of the 41 cities, the coefficient of the purity variable in the regression against the price per gram is positive, with *t* statistics greater than two for 18 of these 32 cities. In 38 of the 41 cities, purity level has a negative effect on price per pure gram; the *t* statistics associated with these coefficients are greater than two in all but one of these cases. For the nine major cities of our data, eight of the nine have positive potency effects on the price per gram and all nine have negative (and significant) potency effects on price per pure gram.

B. Sign and Significance of Potency in Price per Pure Gram Regression* For All Cities

t-value	Negative	Positive
2.00 or more	38	1
less than 2.00	1	1

*$\text{Log}\,(P/SQ) = \beta_0 + \beta_1 \text{Log}\,Q + \beta_2 \text{Log}\,S + \beta_3 \text{Log}\,T.$

Revenue Flows in the Heroin Distribution System

The estimated relation between the price of heroin and the quantity and purity of the purchase can help provide insight into the profitability of the various levels of the distribution system. Table 3 shows the flow of a 30-kilo import of heroin through the distribution system of two cities, New York and Miami. This hypothetical flow is based on an analysis of the New York City heroin market conducted by Mark Moore, 1972a (which borrows heavily from Preble and Casey, 1969).

Moore suggests that there are seven levels of the distribution system from the importer to the addict and that two economic activities may be taking place at each level: dilution of the heroin to a lower level of potency and repackaging into smaller quantities for transactions at the next level. For example, Moore suggests that the importer splits 30 kilograms of heroin into ten three-kilogram lots for sale to the kilo connections. The kilo connections provide two services: they dilute the heroin by half, to a potency level of 40 percent, and they repackage the diluted heroin into one and one-half-kilogram lots for sale to the connections. The connections dilute the heroin again by half, to a potency of 20 percent, and resell the produce in 250-gram lots to the weight dealers.

The final three levels in the distribution system represent levels at which both consumption and sale take place. Moore suggests that the weight dealers dilute the heroin by half and sell the diluted substance in 25-gram lots to the street dealers, who in turn, after consuming 25 percent of the amount they buy, dilute the heroin again to 6 2/3 percent potency and resell it in five-gram packages to the jugglers. Finally, the jugglers, after consuming a third of the heroin they buy, resell the remainder to addicts in quantities of about one gram per transaction. The addicts consume the remainder.

We have used this hypothetical structure of the distribution, along with our analysis, to study the revenue flows in the heroin distribution system. Table 3 summarizes the results of this analysis for New York City and Miami. The rows of this table represent the conditions of the purchase by the individuals at that level. The first five columns represent our interpretation of Moore's analysis of the distribution system. Column 1 represents the total quantity of (diluted) narcotic in the system at the time. Columns 2 and 3 represent the purity level and average lot size of each transaction made at the level. Column 4 represents the number of transactions at that purity and quantity level. Column 5 shows the consumption at each level, which, of course, affects the amount of heroin in the system.

The final three columns are based on our analysis of the structure of the heroin market. Column 7 displays our estimates of the price per gram, given the purity and quantity levels representative of transactions at the various levels of the

Table 3. Estimated Revenue Flows in Heroin Distribution System: New York City and Miami

Level	Total quantity in system at time of purchase (grams)	Purity (percent)	Quantity (grams) Per transaction	Number of transactions	Consumption	Value of consumption	Price per gram (dollars)	Total revenue raised by sales (dollars)
				New York City				
Importer	30,000	80	30,000	1	0	0	15.17	455,100
Kilo Connection	30,000	80	3,000	10	0	0	22.43	672,900
Connection	60,000	40	1,500	40	0	0	20.54	1,232,400
Weight dealers	120,000	20	250	480	0	0	22.63	2,715,600
Street dealers	240,000	10	25	9,600	60,000	1,627,800	27.13	6,511,200
Jugglers	270,000	6.67	5	54,000	90,000	2,846,700	31.63	8,540,100
Addicts	180,000	6.67	1	180,000	180,000	7,486,200	41.59	7,486,200
				Miami				
Importer	30,000	80	30,000	1	0	0	14.19	425,700
Kilo connection	30,000	80	3,000	10	0	0	23.54	706,200
Connection	60,000	40	1,500	40	0	0	23.11	1,386,600
Weight dealers	120,000	20	250	480	0	0	28.84	3,460,800
Street dealers	240,000	10	25	9,600	60,000	2,409,000	40.15	9,636,000
Jugglers	270,000	6.67	5	54,000	90,000	4,659,300	51.77	13,977,900
Addicts	180,000	6.67	1	180,000	180,000	13,280,400	73.78	13,280,400

distribution system. For New York, for example, we estimate a price of $22.43 per gram at the kilo connection level, where heroin is bought 80 percent pure in three-kilo lot sizes; at the juggler level, where heroin is bought at a 6 2/3 percent purity level and in five-gram lot sizes, we estimate a price of $31.63 per gram.

Our price estimates for New York City are quite consistent with those derived by Moore, though his prices are based on an earlier period and do not take into account the quantity and purity effects isolated in this study. The one exception is in the price per gram at the importer level, where Moore suggests a price about a third of the figure we suggest. This discrepancy may, perhaps, be explained by the fact that we have never observed quantities at the 30-kilogram level in our data; the largest purchase is about one-half kilo at about the weight dealer level. Our price estimates at this range may thus not be as accurate as in other ranges. (Our figures, however, are more consistent with those suggested on the BNDD's Form 199 than are Moore's. The report for May 1971, e.g., reports a price range of $16,000 to $27,000 for a kilo of 80-100 percent pure heroin.)

On the basis of our estimated prices, Columns 6 and 8 show the value of consumption at each level of the distribution system and the total revenue raised by sales to that level, respectively. For example, we estimate that in New York the jugglers, who pay a total of about $8.5 million for their heroin, consume about $2.8 million worth and resell the remainder to addicts for about $7.5 million.

Our estimates suggest that the initial 30-kilo import eventually leads to about $12 million in consumption, for an average of $400,000 per kilo, and a total funds flow of nearly $30 million in New York City.

Comparison of the results for New York and Miami suggests an interesting observation. When prices are different in different cities, why do not arbitrage operations take place, with distributors choosing to sell in markets where the price is higher? At the levels of the distribution system in which large quantities of heroin are involved in individual transactions, our price estimates for New York and Miami are very similar—$22.43 per gram versus $23.54 per gram at the kilo connection level, for example, a difference of $3,330 on a three-kilo transaction. It is only at the lower levels of the distribution system, in which the quantity transactions are relatively small, that price-per-gram discrepancies are large.

We estimate that the addicts in New York pay about $42 per gram, while the addicts in Miami pay almost $74 per gram. Because of the smaller transactions at the lower levels, arbitrage operations are probably not profitable due to the costs of transportation and of establishing a distribution system and because of the risk involved; therefore, differences in prices at lower levels may not reflect differences at higher levels.

Time Trends

We had no particular prior opinion about the direction of the time trend because conflicting influences affect the price. For example, general inflation, increasingly strict enforcement of narcotics laws, and a growing number of addicts may lead to increasing prices. On the other hand, the opening of new supply sources (e.g., Vietnam), increases in competition among suppliers, or increasing availability of treatment would tend to lower prices over time. Also, competition among suppliers may drive down prices until one supplier becomes dominant and, through this monopoly power, is able to raise prices.

Of the cities in our data 25 had positive time trends (see Tabulation C), although most of these were not significant. For the major cities, New York, Detroit, Boston and New Orleans had a significant positive trend in price per gram over this time. Almost two-thirds of the cities showed no apparent time trend.

C. Sign and Significance of Time in Price Per Gram Regression* For All Cities

t-value	Negative	Positive
2.00 or more	5	8
less than 2.00	11	17

*$\text{Log}\,(P/Q) = \beta_0 + \beta_1 \text{Log}\,Q + \beta_2 \text{Log}\,S + \beta_3 \text{Log}\,T.$

Stratifying the Heroin Market

A final observation of interest is based on a scatter plot of the quantity and purity of the almost 3,000 heroin buys made in all cities during the two years of our data.

Figure 5 shows that the purchases clustered roughly in three quantity bands: at 0-50 grams, 50-300 grams, and over 400 grams. Within each of these quantity levels, the purity of the purchase spanned the whole range (although there were relatively few large buys less than 30 percent pure). If these buys are at all indicative of the true heroin market (rather than simply the market in which narcotics agents operate), they imply that small-but-potent and large-but-diluted transactions are more common than might have been expected.

The distribution system models of Preble and Casey (1969) and Moore (1972a), discussed earlier, lead to the conclusion that highly potent substances are transacted in large quantities only and that heroin of low potency is transacted in small quantities only. This appears not to be the case. This surprising finding may indicate that free-lance importers selling small quantities of pure heroin without the benefits of a large organization are more common than previously expected.

ANALYSES OF THE RELATIONSHIP BETWEEN DRUG PRICES AND CRIME

The principal reason for constructing these heroin price series is to provide an analytical tool for policy-related studies. Since crime is the externality most frequently associated with the presence of the heroin market, investigations into

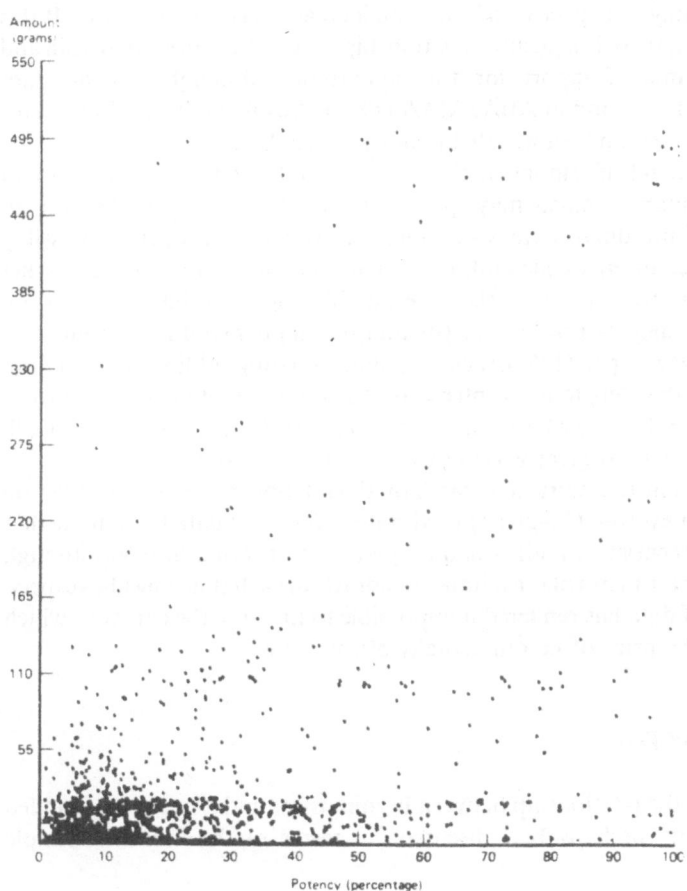

Fig. 5. Plot of Quantity and Potency of Buys in Total Sample

the relationship between heroin prices and the level of crime in various categories are particularly relevant.

Previous Literature

A number of hypotheses may be advanced concerning the possible relations among these variables. For example, if demand for heroin in an area is inelastic, i.e., if addicts must consume a fixed quantity of heroin each period, then, to the extent that addicts support their habit through criminal behavior, a rise in the price of heroin may be expected to lead to an increase in criminal activity. If this hypothesis is true, there is a positive relationship between the price of heroin and the level of crime.[1] Support for this hypothesis, although generally not empirically based, is found in ABA/AMA (1951), Ausubel (1958), Maurer and Vogel (1952), Cohen and Short (1958), and Duvall (1953).

On the other hand, if criminal activity goes on independently of the price of heroin (even though criminals may spend some of their money on heroin), an increase in price presumably causes criminals to consume less heroin, possibly substituting other drugs or alcohol, or moving out of the illicit drug market altogether. When prices are low, they presumably choose to buy more heroin. This hypothesis suggests price-elastic (or unit elastic) demand for heroin.

Kavaler's survey paper (1968) reviews studies relating addiction and criminality. Much of this debate has centered on the direction of causality between criminality and addiction. Maurer and Vogel (1962), Cohen (1958), and Kolb (1965), among others, present varying views on this question.

There has been little empirical research on the relationship between addiction and criminality. Leveson (Chapter 5) used state-aggregated data to estimate that states with 10 percent more addicts had 1.4 percent more crime in 1960, although the quality of the estimates of the number of addicts in each state must be suspect. Unavailability of data has rendered it impossible to measure the extent to which fluctuations in the price of heroin actually affect crime.

Methodology and Data

An analysis of the relationship between heroin prices and crime is confounded by several factors, perhaps best discussed in terms of the following simple relationship:

---

[1]Moore [1972a] estimates that only about 20 percent of the money used to purchase heroin is raised by "street" crime. Other sources are: dealing in the drug (45 percent), prostitution (17 percent), and shoplifting (12 percent).

Total crime = addict crime + non-addict crime
            = crime per addict x the number of addicts
              + non-addict crime.

If addict crime is only a small proportion of the total, statistical isolation of the effects of price fluctuations on total crime statistics may not be possible. This may be the case when the number of addicts in a metropolitan area is small.

A second confounding factor is the discrepancy between the actual level and the reported level of crime. It is generally recognized that crimes in many categories go unreported. In addition, it has been suggested that much criminal activity involves persons or property in the neighborhood known by the criminal (see President's Commission, 1967). If, in fact, much of the addict crime involves other addicts or residents of areas with large addict populations, victims may choose not to report crimes for fear of involvement with the police. Addict crime may thus be systematically underreported, and its proportion of the total crime in a metropolitan area may be underestimated.

The breakdown of addict crime into crime per addict times the number of addicts suggests a further confounding factor. The short- and long-run effects of a high price of heroin on the level of crime may be quite different. For example, in the short run, when the number of addicts and the resulting demand for heroin are relatively fixed, an increase in the price of heroin might lead addicts to higher levels of criminal behavior. On the other hand, high prices for heroin may discourage entry into (and encourage departure from) the addict population and thus lead, in the long run, to a decrease in the number of addicts who commit crime. (Moore [1972b] proposes a pricing scheme for heroin based on this point.) Thus, while high prices of heroin may lead to more crime in the short run, the same high prices may lead to a decrease in crime in the long run as a result of the decrease in the addict population. It is likely that our results pertain to the short-run effects of high prices of heroin; implications from these analyses should be interpreted in this light.

To examine the relationships between price fluctuations and crime, we obtained data from the Federal Bureau of Investigation on reported offenses in each of the major (Part I) categories for our major cities. The Uniform Crime Reports, in addition to the problems with offense data just noted, have the feature that any single incident is classified only in the highest ranking category involved. For example, if an attempted robbery leads to murder, the crime is reported in the category associated with the more severe crime only (in this case, murder).

The categories covered in this reporting system, in decreasing order of precedence, are murder, forcible rape, robbery, aggravated assault, burglary, grand larceny (over \$50), and auto theft. A measure of total crime is obtained by summing the values for the seven categories. We also have data on three additional offense categories; manslaughter, simple assault, and larceny under $50.

A simple model was constructed to relate monthly drug prices and crime:

$$C_t^{(j)} = \beta_0 + \beta_1 (P/Q)_t^* + \beta_2 W_t + \beta_3 t + \epsilon^{(6)}{}_t,$$

where

$C_t^{(j)}$ = reported offenses in Category j in Month t;
$(P/Q)_t^*$ = "retail" price of heroin in Month t;
W_t = average temperature in Month t;
t = month of occurrence.

The parameters of (6) were estimated by ordinary least-squares for each category of offenses for each of the nine cities for which we had the most data. Price estimates for months in which no data were available were obtained by interpolation of adjacent estimates. This was necessary only once for New York City and a few times for other cities.

The temperature and time variables reflect seasonal variations and a trend in the level of crime over the two-year period of the study. Evidence of large seasonality components in offense series is reported by McPheters and Stronge (1972). We do not regard (6) as a final specification of the model relating the price of heroin to crime. Because of such omitted variables as law enforcement, and such alternatives to crime as treatment and substitution into drugs other than heroin, proper estimation of the effects of changes in the heroin market probably necessitates construction of a simultaneous-equations model. Though some demographic variables (e.g., income, education) are certainly related to the incidence of crime, many change very slowly within a city and probably did not change much in the two years under study.

Results for New York City Offenses

The results for the nine major cities are mixed and, in many ways, ambiguous. When the nine cities are viewed together, the estimated relationship between heroin price and crime is unstable. Both positive and negative effects (in some cases, significant) are estimated.

The results for New York City, however, are particularly suggestive of a positive relationship between heroin price and crime. There are two reasons for singling out the New York results. One is that the addict population in New York City is generally recognized to be considerably greater than the addict population in any of the other cities. The conventional wisdom is that half the nation's estimated 150,000-350,000 addicts live in New York (see Wald and Hutt [1972]). For example, Greenwood (1971) estimates 2,800 addicts in Boston, 10,200 in Chicago, 5,500 in New Orleans, and 9,800 in Los Angeles, while estimating 150,000 in New York. (See McGlothlin et al. (1972) and Singer (1971) for alternative estimates.) Thus, addict-related crime is expected to be larger, both absolutely and proportionately, in New York than in other cities.[2]

Second, we have the greatest confidence in our heroin price series for New York City: they are based on 217 observations spread reasonably well over the two-year period.

The estimated crime model for each category of offenses is shown in Table 4. The explanatory power of the model is quite high (about 80 percent) for aggravated assault, grand larceny, and auto theft, and reasonably high for the other categories.

The elasticities of drug price are also shown in Table 4. A positive impact is predicted for eight of the ten crime categories and for the total. Crimes associated with revenue-raising, such as robbery, burglary, larceny, and auto theft, all have predicted positive signs. A 10-percent increase in the price of heroin is predicted to lead to a 3.6-percent increase in robberies, a 1.8-percent increase in burlaries, a 2.0-percent increase in larceny under $50, and a 2.5-percent increase in auto theft. (The t values in each of these categories exceed 1.4.)

The categories not associated with revenue-raising—manslaughter and forcible rape—have estimated t statistics of about 0.1, suggesting that increases in heroin prices are not correlated spuriously with increases in the other crime categories, since there is positive correlation among all eleven crime categories.

The predicted increases in crimes of violence, i.e., murder and aggravated assault, may be attributed either, as has been suggested, to increases in violence within the addict population and distribution system ("...in the last two years, there have been more than 250 murders of middle-level, non-addict heroin and cocaine pushers..." [Pileggi, 1973, p. 34]) as a result of high prices,[3] or to peculiarities in crime-recording. Larger numbers of murders might, in fact, be the result of an increase in robberies, burlaries, and other revenue-raising crimes, some of which lead to murder.

We also estimated models including a (somewhat questionable) monthly series

---

[2]A related hypothesis, suggested by a referee, is that every city supports only a certain number of criminals, and it happens that in New York a relatively larger proportion of the criminals are addicts. The effect of this large number of addict criminals is only a systematic relation between crime and the price of heroin, not an increase in the total amount of crime.

[3]The *Detroit Free Press* of Sept. 4, 1973, reported that 40 percent of the city's homicide victims younger than 35 are under the influence of narcotics when they die. Quoting from the article, "The figures are a stunning new index of the relationship of narcotics and homicide...."

Table 4. Estimated Crime Model for New York*

Crime categories	β_0	β_1	β_2	β_3	R^2	Elasticity
Murder	51.66	1.45 (2.89)	0.04 (0.22)	0.05 (0.07)	0.523	.53
Manslaughter	1.34	0.01 (0.11)	0.03 (0.97)	0.06 (0.59)	0.081	.09
Forcible rape	113.26	0.07 (0.10)	0.81 (3.03)	3.84 (4.11)	0.670	.01
Robbery	6351.3	58.67 (2.24)	−14.18 (−1.40)	−87.84 (−2.48)	0.314	.36
Aggravated assault	1188.3	9.88 (1.73)	19.74 (8.94)	9.52 (1.23)	0.813	.15
Simple assault	2695.0	−17.14 (−1.92)	16.04 (4.65)	14.71 (1.22)	0.607	−.24
Burglary	13251.0	61.19 (1.68)	25.11 (1.79)	-213.05 (−4.33)	0.605	.18
Larceny over $50	9220.7	15.13 (0.51)	49.83 (4.33)	-202.09 (−5.02)	0.806	.06
Larceny under $50	4567.0	22.87 (1.37)	9.39 (1.45)	−92.17 (−4.08)	0.586	.20
Auto theft	6235.3	46.07 (2.38)	26.58 (3.55)	-157.92 (−6.04)	0.771	.25
Index total	36412.0	192.48 (1.83)	107.93 (2.66)	-647.50 (−4.56)	0.655	.19

*$C_t = \beta_0 + \beta_1 (P/Q)_t{}^* + \beta_2 (\text{temp.})_t + \beta_3 (\text{time})_t$

on unemployment. The results led to somewhat higher drug price elasticities and t-statistics in the revenue-related crime categories, but also to implausible signs on the unemployment variable, although empirical evidence of the effect of unemployment on crime is not supportive of any particular sign (see Philips, et al., 1972).[4]

Taxicab Robberies

A further piece of analysis, again based on data from New York City, lends support to the conclusions obtained from analysis of the Uniform Crime

---

[4]We note in passing that there is considerably more assault, larceny, and auto theft in warm months and somewhat more robberies in cold months.

Reports. As noted previously, one of the problems in use of offense data is the potential underreporting of crimes, particularly of crimes committed by addicts. We obtained New York City data concerning the number of taxicab robberies, offenses said to be fully reported. The same model (6) was estimated to relate the number of taxicab robberies to the price of heroin. The results are:

Number of robberies
$$= 301.25 + 0.78\,(P/Q)^* + 0.45W - 12.61t \qquad R^2 = 0.77,$$
$$\ \ (4.2)\quad (0.5)\qquad\qquad (0.7)\qquad (-5.4)$$

Value of robberies
$$= 11569.7 + 27.02\,(P/Q)^* + 17.25W - 490.45t \quad R^2 = 0.72.$$
$$\ \ (3.6)\quad (0.4)\qquad\qquad (0.6)\qquad (-4.8)$$

Higher prices of heroin are associated with an increase in both the number and total yield of taxicab robberies, although the t statistics associated with these coefficients are not large. The estimated elasticities of the number of robberies and the yield of taxicab robberies are 0.17 and 0.16, respectively. (The average yield per robbery was probably unaffected, as seems reasonable.) Thus, a 10-percent increase in the price of heroin is predicted to lead to an increase of 1.7-percent in the number of taxicab robberies each month.

Results for Other Cities

The results for New York City are indicative of a positive short-run relationship between the price of heroin and the level of crime in revenue-raising categories. As we noted earlier, the results for the other eight major cities are not generally in accord with these conclusions. For some cities (e.g., Houston), we find a positive relationship between drug prices and crime; for other cities (e.g., Boston), we find a significant negative relationship. In Chicago, Detroit and Miami, both positive and negative signs are estimated, although none of the t statistics associated with the drug price coefficient are large.

It is likely that a systematic investigation of the relationship between drug prices and crime is confounded by the likelihood that addict-related crime is small relative to the total and by the paucity of price data for some of the relevant cities.

We feel, however, that this preliminary work is highly suggestive, not only of a short-run positive relationship between drug prices and crime, but also of the type of research that can be conducted through such statistics as those developed in this chapter. For a more recent treatment of the crime-heroin price relationship, see Silverman and Spruill (1977).

ACKNOWLEDGEMENTS

This paper appeared in the *J. Am. Stat. Assoc.* (1974) *69* (347): 595-606, and as a Drug Abuse Council monograph. The permission of the Association and the Council to reprint are appreciated. Support for the study was provided by the Drug Abuse Council; data were provided by the Bureau of Narcotics and Dangerous Drugs (now Drug Enforcement Administration). Research assistance was performed by Dale Wanderer. The authors wish to thank Paul Feldman, Stan Horowitz, and Chris Jehn of the Center for Naval Analyses, and Jim DeLong and John Sessler of the Drug Abuse Council for helpful discussions and comments.

REFERENCES

American Bar Association and American Medical Association, Joint Committee on Narcotic Drugs, *Drug Addiction: Crime or Disease?* Bloomington, Ind.: Indiana University Press, 1961.

Ausubel, David P., "Causes and types of narcotic addiction, a psycho-social view," *Psychiatric Quarterly,* 35 (July 1961), 523-31.

Ausubel, David P., *Drug Addiction: Physiological, Psychological, and Sociological Aspects,* New York: Random House, 1958.

Brown, George F., Jr. and Silverman, Lester P., "The Retail Price of Heroin: Estimation and Applications," Public Research Institute, PRI 73-1, March 1973.

Cohen, Albert K. and Short, James F., "Research in delinquent subcultures," *Journal of Social Issues,* 14, No. 3 (1958), 20-37.

Committee on Government Operations of the U.S. Senate, "Organized Crime and Illicit Traffic in Narcotics," Washington, D.C., U.S. Government Printing Office, 1965.

Duvall, H.J., "Follow-up study of narcotic drug addicts five years after hospitalization," *Public Health Reports,* 78 (March 1953), 185-93.

Greenwood, Joseph A., "Estimating number of narcotic addicts," Bureau of Narcotics and Dangerous Drugs, Washington, D.C., October 1971.

Kavaler, Florence, "A commentary and annotated bibliography on the relationship between narcotics addiction and criminality," *Municipal Reference Library Notes,* 62, No. 4 (April 1968), 45-63.

Kolb, Lawrence, *Drug Addiction, A Medical Problem,* Springfield, Ill.: Charles C. Thomas, 1962.

Kolb, Lawrence, "Drug addiction in its relation to crime," *Mental Hygiene,* 9 (January 1925), 74-89.

Maurer, D.W. and Vogel, V.H., *Narcotics and Narcotic Addiction,* 2nd ed., Springfield, Ill.: Charles C. Thomas, 1962.

McGlothlin, William H., "Alternative Approaches to Opiate Addiction Control: Costs, Benefits and Potential," Final Report, BNDD Contract No. J-70-33, June 1972.

McPheters, Lee R. and Stronge, William B., "Testing for Seasonality on Reported Crime Data," Working paper, Florida Atlantic University; presented to ORSA Meeting, Atlantic City, November 1972.

Moore, Mark, "Economics of heroin distribution," *Policy Concerning Drug Abuse in New York State, Vol. 3:* Croton-on-Hudson, N.Y.: Hudson Institute, Inc., July 20, 1972.

Moore, Mark, "Law Enforcement to Achieve Discrimination on the Effective Price of Heroin," Working paper, presented to American Economic Association, Toronto, December 1972.

Philips, L., Votey, H.L. and Maxwell, D., "Crime, youth, and the labor market," *Journal of Political Economy,* 80, No. 3, Part I (May/June 1972), 491-504.

Pileggi, Nicholas, "Anatomy of the drug war," *New York,* Jan. 8, 1973, 33-39.

Preble, Edward and Casey, John J., Jr., "Taking care of business—The heroin user's life on the street," *International Journal of the Addictions,* 4, No. 1 (March 1969), 1-24.

President's Commission on Law Enforcement and Administration of Justice, "The Challenge of Crime in a Free Society," Washington, D.C.: U.S. Government Printing Office, February 1967.

Redlinger, L.J., *Dealing in Dope: Market Mechanisms and Distribution Patterns of Illicit Narcotics,* Ann Arbor, Mich.: University Microfilsm, Inc., 1970.

Rottenberg, Simon, "The clandestine distribution of heroin, its discovery and suppression," *Journal of Political Economy,* 76, No. 1 (January/February 1968), 78-90.

Silverman, Lester P. and Spruill, Nancy L., "Urban Crime and the Price of Heroin," *Journal of Urban Economics,* 4, 80–103, 1977.

Singer, Max, "The vitality of mythical numbers," *The Public Interest,* 3, No. 23 (Spring 1971), 3-9.

Wald, Patricia M. and Hutt, Peter Barton, *Dealing with Drug Abuse,* New York: Praeger Publishers, 1972.

CHAPTER 4

The Impact of Drug Addiction on Criminal Earnings

DOUGLAS COATE
FRED GOLDMAN

One of the overwhelming reasons for public concern with the consumption of heroin and other illicit drugs is the presumed impact of their use on criminal activity. Heroin addicts in particular have been held responsible for much of the crime that is committed in urban America, although there are a variety of numbers attached to the word "much" (Casey and Preble, 1974; Patch, 1973; Singer, 1971). Although nearly every researcher of the drug use/crime nexus has established that consumers of illicit drugs commit income-generating criminal acts (Greenberg and Adler, 1974), no one has established the direction and extent of this relationship.[1] Yet, knowledge of the amount of crime stimulated by drug consumption is vital for effective allocation of law enforcement resources and for equitable formulation of legal sanctions against drug consumption and distribution. The purpose of this paper is to develop empirical estimates of the extent to

---

[1]Brown and Silverman (Chapter 3) and Silverman and Spruill (1975) provide empirical estimates of the impact of changes over time in a "heroin price index" on total criminal offenses reported to the police in a given city. The offenses do not distinguish between addict and non-addict crime, however, and it is not obvious how to interpret findings based on the index. For a discussion of these and related papers see Goldman (1976).

which the consumption of heroin and other illicit drugs lead to income-generating criminal activity. We particularly emphasize the relationship between drug expenditures and earnings from crimes other than drug selling.[2]

PREVIOUS LITERATURE

The theoretical structures of past research on the relationship between drug consumption and criminal activity have been incomplete. Previous investigators have omitted from their theoretical constructs at least one of the following aspects of the drug use/criminal activity decision: 1) the simultaneous determination of drug expenditures and criminal activity; 2) the income accruing to drug users/sellers from drug distribution; 3) the existence of legal employment opportunities for drug users. We now turn to a brief discussion of these considerations.

Virtually all past research on the relationship between drug consumption and criminal activity assumes that causality runs solely from drug use to participation in criminal activity. Casey and Preble (1974, pp. 283–307), for example, estimate the dollar costs of crime resulting from the use of narcotic drugs by substracting both an approximation of the dollar cost of subsistence living and an estimate of legal earnings from their estimate of total drug expenditures by the nation's "addict" population. A similar approach is suggested by Holahan (1972, pp. 255–299). Although drug use may be a motivating force for some income-generating crime, causality may also run in the reverse direction. To put this quite simply income should be an important determinant of drug expenditures.

The fact that many drug dealers are also users implies that a portion of drug consumption is financed by funds generated within the distribution network. For instance, Hughes et al. (1971) observed a "heroin copping community" where 34 percent of the 125 addicts were primarily engaged in drug distribution and Moore (1970) has estimated that 50 percent of the monies spent on heroin are obtained from drug sales and the sale of related services. Holahan (1972, p. 289) presents evidence that persons who consume relatively large quantities of heroin tend to be drug dealers. Thus, even if one took the extreme view that drug use forced participation in illegal markets to completely finance drug expenditures, it would not follow that income from crimes against persons and property would approximate the value of drug consumption.

Drug selling and nondrug crime are not the only sources of funds for financing drug use. Hughes (1971, p. 46) found that users in legal occupations "who reported less frequent use and less expensive habits, paid for their drugs largely through their own legitimate income." The National Commission on Marijuana

---

[2]These crimes are primarily against persons and property.

and Drug Abuse (1973), after an extensive review of the literature relating drug addiction and criminal behavior, reports that 41 to 66 percent of the various study populations were employed immediately prior to arrest, incarceration, or treatment.

SPECIFICATION OF THE MODEL

The previous discussion suggests that the relationship between illicit drug use and participation in criminal activity should be analyzed within the context of a model that would also include drug selling income and legal income as endogenous variables. We specify such a model in Table 1 and Figure 1. It consists for four structural equations and four endogenous or jointly determined variables.[3] The jointly determined variables are income from the selling of drugs (S), income from all crime except drug selling (C), income from legal activities (L), and dollar size of drug consumption (D). The drug expenditure coefficient in the nondrug criminal earnings equation (equation 1, Table 1) will indicate the change in income from nondrug crime that results from a dollar increase in drug consumption. The estimation of this relationship is the central focus of this paper. Next, we briefly discuss the composition of each of the structural equations of the model as shown in Table 1 and diagrammed in Figure 1.

The Determinants of Income from Nondrug Crimes (Equation 1) and the Determinants of Income from Drug Sales (Equation 2)

We hypothesize that the addict's income from nondrug crimes (C) is a function of expenditures on drugs (D), income from legal employment (L), income from the selling of drugs (S) and other socioeconomic and family background variables which may influence the addict's calculation of the "costs" and "benefits" of engaging in criminal activity. The determinants of the addict's income from drug selling are hypothesized to be similar explanatory variables. In this equation, income from nondrug crimes replaces income from drug selling as a right hand side (endogenous) variable. The dollar size of habit coefficient (D) in each of the criminal activity equations will indicate the change in income from either drug selling or nondrug crimes that results from a dollar increase in drug habit.

Legal earnings (L) are also included in the criminal activity equations as an

---

[3]"Endogenous" or "jointly determined variables" are determined within the model. "Exogenous" variables are "predetermined," or determined outside of the model.

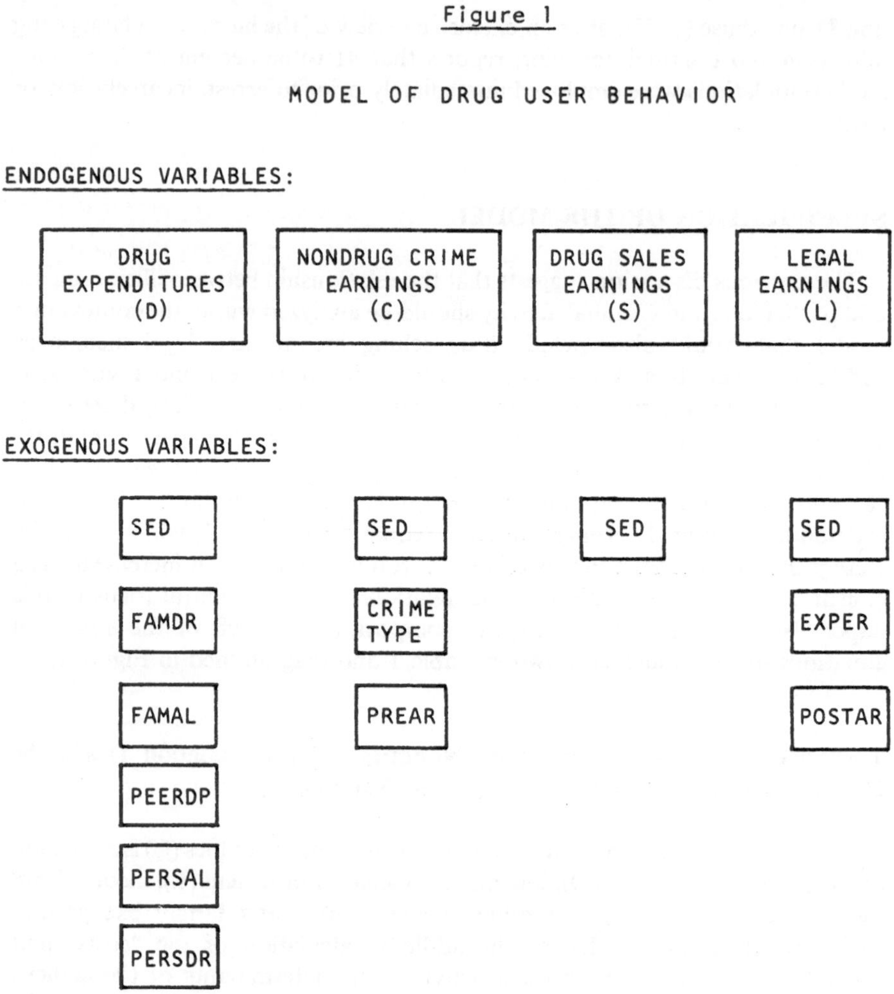

Figure 1

MODEL OF DRUG USER BEHAVIOR

ENDOGENOUS VARIABLES:

| DRUG EXPENDITURES (D) | NONDRUG CRIME EARNINGS (C) | DRUG SALES EARNINGS (S) | LEGAL EARNINGS (L) |

EXOGENOUS VARIABLES:

SED	SED	SED	SED
FAMDR	CRIME TYPE		EXPER
FAMAL	PREAR		POSTAR
PEERDP			
PERSAL			
PERSDR			

Fig. 1. Model of Drug User Behavior

Table 1. Econometric Model of Drug User Behavior*

$C = c\ (\hat{D}, \hat{S}, \hat{L}, \hat{V}_1)$	(1)
$S = s\ (\hat{D}, \hat{C}, \hat{L}, \hat{V}_2)$	(2)
$L = l\ (\hat{D}, \hat{C}, \hat{S}, \hat{V}_3)$	(3)
$D = d\ (\hat{C}, \hat{S}, \hat{L}, \hat{V}_4)$	(4)

*V_1, V_2, V_3, V_4, are vectors of exogenous variables identified in figure 1. A carat (ˆ) over a variable indicates that it is endogenous.

endogenous variable. Generally, increases in legal earnings should bring about reductions in criminal activity. This is because part of the costs of devoting time to criminal activity is the legal income which is foregone. Even if addicts engage in criminal activities at times when their legal earnings opportunities are very small, increases in legal earnings *raise* the costs of engaging in criminal activity. This is because incarceration may preclude the continuation of legal earnings. Moreover, the decrease in criminal activity should be relatively greater among higher risk crimes. Other things equal, the rational addict would choose smaller amounts of crime in response to increases in its cost. It is also expected that dollars gained from drug selling and from nondrug crimes are substitutes and will be inversely related in the estimated criminal activity equations.

Socioeconomic and demographic factors are also expected to influence the amount of criminal activity engaged in by addicts. Brief discussions of their probable effects are listed below.

Age

Literature cited above suggests that as addicts age they mature out of drug use and the criminal lifestyle and conform to more conventional behavior. Drug use and crime would be expected to increase with age to a point and then decrease. This relationship is represented by a parabola. It is estimated by entering both age and the square of age into the criminal activity and drug expenditures equations.

Schooling

The effect of schooling on criminal activity is uncertain. Schooling may make the addict a more efficient and successful criminal in the same way it serves to make him more productive in legal markets. On the other hand, higher levels of schooling may imply a greater opportunity to gain more satisfactory employment (in a psychological sense), holding legal income constant. This should discourage the addict's participation in criminal activities.

Ethnicity

Ehrlich (1974) has found differences in crime patterns by race after controlling for other variables. He concludes that non-whites commit more crimes than whites because they have less opportunity in legal markets while, at the same time, they have equal opportunity in illegal ones.

Criminal History

A review of the literature reveals strong support for the hypothesis that many addicts are of the "type" who engage in criminal activity prior to addiction (Goldman, 1976). That is, prior to addiction, the evaluation of these persons of their opportunities in legal and illegal markets and their attitudes toward risk resulted in their participation in criminal activities. Some investigators suggest that addicts are faced with basically the same choices during their addicted years and, thus, choose an amount of criminal activity that is not significantly influenced by their drug use. Therefore, to properly estimate the extent of the relationship running from drug addiction to criminal activity, the criminal activities that result from facing an array of choices similar to those of the years prior to addiction should be separated from those criminal activities which occur because of the need to secure drugs. This is accomplished, in part, by including the socioeconomic variables in the criminal activity equation. The age variable, for example, would control for the likelihood that younger addicts choose to engage in more criminal activities which do not result from the need for drugs than do older addicts.

It is possible to further control for the criminal activity that results for reasons other than the need to secure drugs. This is done by entering into the equations variables that describe the addict's pre-addiction criminal activity. Addicts with higher rates of pre-addiction criminal activity may be more likely to engage in post-addiction illegal activity. These addicts have already demonstrated that the array of opportunities they face, independent of any need for drugs, results in their choice of higher rates of participation in illegal markets.

The Determinants of Legal Earnings (Equation 3)

The determinants of the legal earnings of addicts (L) are analyzed in equation 3. The remaining three endogenous variables, dollar size of habit (D) and income from drug selling (S) and nondrug crime (C) appear as independent variables in this equation.

The effect of drug expenditures on legal earnings is not obvious, *a priori*. Increases in the dollar size of habit should increase the need for monies. Holding income from criminal activity constant, it is reasonable to expect the addict to increase his legal earnings. On the other hand, size of habit could be inversely related to legal earnings if increases in habit adversely affect legal market productivity. This situation is more likely to hold in legal markets than illegal markets because in illegal markets the addict is likely to be "self-employed" where as his legal market activities are likely to be monitored.

Income from criminal activity should be inversely related to legal earnings. An increase in illegal income increases the opportunity cost of engaging in legal market activity and could also result in an increased purchase of leisure time.

Work experience and education are included in equation 3 because both enhance legal market earnings by increasing the productivity of the worker.

The criminal record of the addict is expected to have a pejorative effect on addict employment opportunities and, hence, on legal earnings. Potential employers are likely to be reluctant to hire persons with criminal records. To capture this effect as a determinant of legal earnings we employ a series of pre-addiction and post-addiction criminal record variables. Although we expect them to be inversely related to legal earnings, this may not strictly be the case if potential employers are unaware of past criminal activity.

The remaining independent variables are the same socioeconomic and demographic variables which appeared in equation 1. The importance of controlling for race, sex and religion in income-generating functions has been well established (see Juster, 1975; Welch, 1973; Fuchs, 1971).

The Determinants of Weekly Drug Expenditures (Equation 4)

Income from nondrug criminal activity (C) and drug sales (S) appear as endogenous variables in the dollar size of habit equation. We hypothesize that they will be positively associated with drug expenditure. The only implication of this hypothesis is that heroin and other drugs are "normal" goods—other things equal, an increase in income should lead to an increase in expenditures on them. By the same argument, the other endogenous variable in the equation, legal earnings, should also be positively associated with drug expenditures.

Explanations of variation in the dollar size of habit go beyond the purely economic. Wurmser (1972), for example, has characterized the etiology of drug dependence as a series of concentric rings where "the innermost circle is the individual's own deeper problems, the next circle is the family, the third the peer group, the fourth the society-at-large, the fifth the culture and its values, and the sixth and farthest out, the philosophical problem of human existence" (Wurmser, 1972, p.394). This suggests the need to control for the influence of background variables which "predispose" individuals toward drug use. Entered into equation 4 are the use of alcohol and drugs by family members, the use of drugs by peers, the individual's pre-addiction use of drugs and alcohol, as well as the socioeconomic and demographic characteristics of the individual.

THE DATA AND STATISTICAL TECHNIQUES

The model is estimated by two-stage least squares regression analysis using data derived from the 1970 Phoenix House Survey of the addict population residing in Phoenix House therapeutic communities between July 1970 and

July 1971. Definitions of the variables which were statistically significant and part of the second stage estimates are presented in Figure 1.[4]

MEASUREMENT OF ENDOGENOUS VARIABLES

Two of the endogenous variables, earnings from nondrug crime (C) and drug expenditures (D), are measured for the same week. A weakness in the data is that the legal income variable, salary at last job (L), is not necessarily specific to this same week. It is not clear how many persons were employed at their last job in that week for which D and C were reported. There is evidence, previously cited, that addict employment rates are as high as 66 percent. The Phoenix House data are also consistent with the hypothesis of relatively high employment levels for drug users. Eighty-five percent of the sample had worked at a job for a month or more and nearly 80 percent of this subsample reported they worked while on drugs. Nevertheless, we can not be sure what portion of the sample were employed and earning their salary at their last job in that week for which D and C were reported.

A similar problem exists with the measure of drug sale income (S). This variable was reported as drug sale income "usually made per week." We do not know how closely "usual" drug cale income approximates the drug sale income of that week for which the size of habit and nondrug crime figures were reported. Since our major goal in this paper is to determine the impact of drug expenditures on nondrug criminal earnings, three different behavioral models are estimated in this paper to test the sensitivity of this relationship to the data limitations just described. The formal model is reduced to equations 1 and 4 in one set of estimates by eliminating the legal income and drug sale income variables. Although this ensures that the remaining endogenous variables are time specific, the assumptions that legal earnings and drug sale income of the

---

[4]Our behavioral hypotheses cannot be tested by means of ordinary least squares regression analysis. This is because causality runs back to the independent variables when our endogenous variables are included as dependent variables in the specified equations. The statistical problem presented by this interdependency can be overcome if two-stage least squares is used as the estimating technique. In the first stage of this procedure, predicted values for the endogenous variables are obtained by regressing each endogenous variable against all the exogenous variables in the model. In the second stage the structural equations are estimated by ordinary least squares after the predicted values of endogenous variables are substituted for their true values in those equations where they appear as independent variables.

Many of the independent variables which were expected to play an important role in the model turned out to be statistically insignificant when the model was estimated. These variables appear in Figure 1 but are not present in the second-stage estimates shown below.

user are zero or uncorrelated with remaining right hand side variables are required.[5] For the second set of estimates, the legal income equation is added to the two equation model. This model is based on the assumption that drug sale income is zero for the week of heaviest non-drug sale criminal activity or uncorrelated with right hand side variables and that all persons were earning the salary from their last job. Finally, the complete four-equation model is estimated as shown in Table 1.

Although terms such as "addict" and "drug abuser" are usually taken to indicate heroin use, drug dependence[6] is not limited to heroin. Many treatment programs, for example, admit persons "addicted" to a variety of amphetamines, barbiturates and hallucinogens. Since the drug/crime problem is often interpreted solely as a heroin/crime problem, we have estimated the model over a subsample restricted to heroin addicts. However, we have also estimated the model over the entire sample of drug users. These latter set of estimates contain the dummy variable Heroin Addiction to control for the differential impact that heroin may have as compared to other drugs.

THE EMPIRICAL RESULTS

The second stage estimates of all models are presented in Tables 2–5. In our discussion of the empirical results we emphasize the relationship between drug expenditures and nondrug criminal earnings.

Nondrug Criminal Earnings Equations

The second-stage estimates of the Nondrug Criminal Earnings equation are shown in Table 2. The coefficient of Drug Expenditures in the nondrug criminal

---

[5]The bias in the estimated coefficients caused by omitting these variables will depend upon the product of the partial effect of the omitted variable on the dependent variable and the correlations between the independent and omitted variables. Since the three- and four-equation models are estimated, the direction and extent of the bias can be observed by comparing the coefficients in each model. However, we are still left with the problem that legal earnings and drug sale earnings may not be time specific with the week of reported crime and drug use. It is this potential for bias, the relationship between the *actual* legal and drug sale earnings at that time and our proxies, that remain unobserved and indeterminate.

[6]Drug dependence and "addiction" are not well understood. They involve the interrelated issues of psysiological dependency, psychological dependency and the pharmacological properties of the given drug. For an extensive review of this literature see J. DeLong (1972).

earnings equations ranges from 0.45 in the two-equation model to 0.28 in the four-equation model. These estimates are generally highly significant. The ranges are quite different, however, for the set of estimates for all drugs of addiction and those for heroin. A $1.00 increase in heroin addiction, specifically, leads to an 18–29 cent increase in criminal earnings, with the estimate of the impact of heroin use on crime declining as additional sources of income are accounted for. That is, a $1.00 increase in heroin consumption leads to an amount of nondrug sale crime that nets 29 cents in the two-equation model. With legal earnings accounted for (three-equation model) it is reduced to 27 cents. When earnings from drug sales

Table 2. Criminal Earnings*

| | Two Equation Model | | | |
| | All Drugs of Addiction | | Heroin | |
Independent Variables†	Regression Coefficient	Adjusted t-Value	Regression Coefficient	Adjusted t-Value
Drug Expenditures	0.445	4.71	0.287	2.70
Legal Earnings				
Sale of Drugs Earnings				
Pimp/Prostitute	50.931	1.95	60.930	2.15
Prostitute	81.164	−2.61	−69.245	−2.17
Other Illegal Acts	−32.788	−1.78	−24.792	−1.23
Heroin Addiction	−44.779	−2.35		
Constant	65.64	2.98	60.86	2.34
Sample Size	N = 998		N = 802	

* See Table 1 for definitions of variables.
† A carat (ˆ) over a variable indicates that it is endogenous.

Table 2. (cont.) Criminal Earnings

| | Three Equation Model* | | | |
| | All Drugs of Addiction | | Heroin | |
Independent Variables†	Regression Coefficient	Adjusted t-Value	Regression Coefficient	Adjusted t-Value
Drug Expenditures	0.386	3.73	0.272	2.45
Legal Earnings	0.244	0.86	0.111	0.37
Sale of Drugs Earnings				
Pimp/Prostitute	53.486	2.07	60.542	2.15
Prostitute	−71.637	−2.18	−65.054	−1.92
Other Illegal Acts	−28.359	−1.54	−23.983	−1.19
Heroin Addiction	−42.772	−2.26		
Constant	55.63	2.09	54.15	1.76
Sample Size	N = 998		N = 802	

* See Table 1 for definitions of variables.
† A carat (ˆ) over a variable indicates that it is endogenous.

Table 2. Criminal Earnings

| Independent Variables† | Two Equation Model* | | | |
| | All Drugs of Addiction | | Heroin | |
	Regression Coefficient	Adjusted t-Value	Regression Coefficient	Adjusted t-Value
Drug Expenditures	0.445	4.71	0.287	2.70
Legal Earnings				
Sale of Drugs Earnings				
Pimp/Prostitute	50.931	1.95	60.930	2.15
Prostitute	81.164	−2.61	−69.245	−2.17
Other Illegal Acts	−32.788	−1.78	−24.792	−1.23
Heroin Addiction	−44.779	−2.35		
Constant	65.64	2.98	60.86	2.34
Sample Size	N = 998		N = 802	

* See Table 1 for definitions of variables.

† A carat ⁽ˆ⁾ over a variable indicates that it is endogenous.

are included the impact is further reduced to 18 cents and the statistical significance of this coefficient falls markedly.

The estimates based upon users of any drug of addiction range from 28–45 cents. In each of these models the Drug Expenditures coefficient is *larger* than its counterpart estimated over the heroin subsample and declines as additional sources of income are accounted for. Moreover, the criminal earnings of persons whose addiction was to heroin averages about $45 *less* than the criminal earnings of persons addicted to drugs other than heroin. This finding is significant in the two- and three-equation models. In the four-equation model the coefficient on the Heroin Addiction dummy is $20 and the t-statistic falls to below 1.0.

These findings provide support for the hypothesis that illicit drug use leads to nondrug crime. However, there is no support in these results for the extreme view that drug use causes "addicts" to engage in crimes against persons or property that result in income approximately equal to the value of drug expenditures. In fact, when all income sources are accounted for, the drug expenditure effect on nondrug crime appears to be relatively small. Moreover, the parameter estimates imply that the effect of drug expenditures is *smaller* for heroin users than for users of other drugs. And, despite their larger drug expenditures, the nondrug criminal earnings of heroin users are not significantly different from those addicted to other drugs.

Legal earnings and, then, earnings from drug sales are assumed to be endogenous and enter the criminal earnings equation in the 3 and 4 equation models, respectively. The coefficients of these variables do not approach statistical significance. These results are unexpected. Increases in earnings from either of these sources should lead to decreases in nondrug crime, either because of an increase in opportunity cost or because of an increased purchase of leisure time.

Table 3. Drug Expenditures

| | Two Equation Model* | | | |
| | All Drugs of Addiction | | Heroin | |
Independent Variables†	Regression Coefficient	Adjusted t-Value	Regression Coefficient	Adjusted t-Value
Criminal Earnings	0.971	2.94	1.212	2.97
Legal Earnings				
Sale of Drugs Earnings				
Age	21.186	2.191	25.854	2.52
Age squared	−0.251	−1.62	−0.319	−1.85
Months Before Mainlining	−0.569	−1.78	−0.840	−1.66
Female	63.886	3.07	59.015	2.37
Heroin Addiction	55.245	2.12		
Constant	−259.2	−2.38	−302.4	−2.40
Sample Size	N = 998		N = 802	

* See Table 1 for definitions of variables.
† A carat (ˆ) over a variable indicates that it is endogenous.

Table 3. (cont.) Drug Expenditures

| | Three Equation Model* | | | |
| | All Drugs of Addiction | | Heroin | |
Independent Variables†	Regression Coefficient	Adjusted t-Value	Regression Coefficient	Adjusted t-Value
Criminal Earnings	0.778	2.90	0.889	3.16
Legal Earnings	−0.462	−1.15	−0.494	−1.14
Sale of Drugs Earnings				
Age	30.812	3.20	35.238	3.57
Age squared	−0.387	−2.47	−0.446	−2.70
Months Before Mainlining	−0.591	−1.98	−0.677	−1.58
Female	59.908	2.90	52.765	2.28
Heroin Addiction	48.482	2.03		
Constant	−325.8	−3.12	355.1	3.13
Sample Size	N = 998		N = 802	

* See Table 1 for definitions of variables.
† A carat (ˆ) over a variable indicates that it is endogenous.

Table 3. (cont.) Drug Expenditures

| | Four Equation Model* | | | |
| | All Drugs of Addiction | | Heroin | |
Independend Variables†	Regression Coefficient	Adjusted d-Value	Regression Coefficient	Adjusted t-Value
Criminal Earnings	0.890	2.56	0.871	2.46
Legal Earnings	-0.654	-1.17	-0.784	-1.31
Sale of Drugs Earnings	0.214	2.46	0.217	2.28
Age	24.188	2.03	30.918	2.59
Age squared	-0.355	-1.83	-0.434	2.17
Months Before Mainling	-0.257	0.62	-0.006	-0.01
Female	16.883	0.62	21.275	0.69
Heroin Addiction	49.016	1.65		
Constant	-272.7	-2.07	-324.6	-2.39
Sample Size	N = 801		N = 653	

* See Table 1 for definitions of variables.

† A carat (ˆ) over a variable indicates that it is endogenous.

Drug Expenditures (D)

The second-stage estimates of the Drug Expenditures equation are shown in Table 3. The coefficient on criminal earnings ranges from 0.78–1.21 and is significant at the one-percent level in all three models. This indicates that nearly all of a $1.00 increase in nondrug criminal earnings is spent on drugs.[7] This result and the findings previously discussed imply a different explanation of addict behavior than that commonly offered. The observation that drug addicts engage in income-producing crimes against persons and property and use much of those funds to finance drug consumption is consistent with the drug expenditure equation results. However, the motivation for the criminal behavior does not seem to be the need for drugs.

A reasonable scenario, and one which is supported by these empirical results, is that the typical drug user's opportunities in legal and illegal markets and his attitudes toward risk and other related considerations dictate some participation in criminal activities. The delinquent lifestyle may then provide ready contact with drugs and drug users. Drug consumption and illegal activity then become intertwined, although causality for the most part runs from illegal activity to drug

---

[7]The single instance where the marginal propensity to consume heroin out of criminal earnings is $1.21 implies that the consumption of other goods and services is reduced by 21 cents for every dollar increase in criminal earnings, and one dollar plus the 21 cents is spent on heroin. The anecdotal literature on the drug user's lifestyle lends credence to finds of a marginal propensity to consume of approximately unity.

use. This is consistent with the fact that many methadone patients, despite elimination of the need for heroin, still actively engage in criminal activities. This suggests that substantial reductions in the available supply of heroin and other narcotic drugs may not result in substantial fall offs in crimes against persons and property.[8]

The above argument must be tentative. Although the coefficients of most of the exogenous variables specified in the models were highly significant and of the expected sign and magnitude,[9] results which lend further credence to our findings, the relationships among the endogenous legal and illegal income variables, however, were not as hypothesized. This problem has already been discussed in the case of the nondrug crime equation. It reoccurs in another form in the drug expenditure equation. Legal earnings are inversely related to drug expenditures. Also, the drug sale income effect on drug expenditures is not nearly so great as the nondrug crime effect. One explanation for the finding that increases in legal income result in reductions in drug expenditures is that the "costs" of continued drug use increase with legal income and this increase in cost out-weighs any positive effect of income on drug consumption. The cost of drug use would increase with legal income if discovery of drug use by the employer would lead to dismissal or, perhaps, a reduction in earnings. This "cost effect" is not as relevant to illegal market activities where self employment predominates. This would explain why the income effect dominates in the case of increases in illegal income. Another explanation of these results is that drug sellers price discriminate against employed drug users in an attempt to charge what the market will bear. Persons engaged in legal market activities are not "on the street" and information concerning drug markets may be less readily available to them.

The results from the drug sale equations indicate that a $1.00 increase in drug expenditures leads to a $1.50 increase in drug selling income. Our explanation of this result is more statistical than behavioral. Drug sale income "usually made" is likely to substantially overstate the drug sale income actually made during the week of reported drug expenditures and nondrug crime. If this is true, the drug sale income coefficient in the drug expenditure equation would be downward biased and the drug expenditure coefficient in the drug selling equation would be upward biased. As we indicated earlier, the drug sale coefficient was smaller than expected in the drug expenditures equation.

---

[8]Irving Lukoff (1973) has offered a similar hypothesis after the study of inner city drug users enrolled in a New York City methadone maintenance program.

[9]We do not present a discussion of the roles of the exogenous variables in the behavioral models. Some of the exogenous effects considered are: the returns to illegal activity by type of crime; the effects of age on illegal activity and drug consumption (tests of the "maturing out" hypothesis); sex differences in drug expenditures and earnings; and the legal returns to schooling for drug users. These may be derived from the results shown in Tables 2-5.

A final result is worthy of discussion. Drug expenditures are negatively related to legal income. This finding is consistent with the hypothesis that drug use has a debilitating effect on worker productivity. Since commitment to the labor force (Full-time-Worker dummy) and drug use on the job (Worked-While-on-Drugs dummy) are being controlled, it is difficult to argue that this result could be explained by "heavier" drug users seeking out less intensive employment.

CONCLUSIONS

Literature on the nature of drug abuse is in a state of flux. We now know that heroin use need not *irreversibly* lead to heroin addiction. New words enter the drug researcher's lexicon—*chipper, weekender* and *intermittant* or *occassional user*—and all appear to be stable patterns of use which are easily supported by legal activities. Similarly, one must question whether drug abuse must lead, irreversibly, to criminal activities. We have found evidence that the impact of drug abuse on criminal activities is considerably more muted than earlier, impressionistic statements would suggest. In fact, it is the opposite relationship, one in which criminal earnings are spent on drugs of abuse, that appears to dominate the interdependency between drug use and crime. The impact of drug use on criminal activity is further reduced as other sources of income—income from drug selling and legal market activities—are accounted for.

Table 4. Legal Earnings

| Independent Variables† | Three Equation Model* | | | |
| | All Drugs of Addiction | | Heroin | |
	Regression Coefficient	Adjusted t-Value	Regression Coefficient	Adjusted t-Value
Criminal Earnings	0.121	1.78	0.129	1.56
Sale of Drugs Earnings				
Drug Expenditures	0.045	1.31	0.038	0.97
Age	–0.572	–1.05	–0.516	–0.88
Time At Longest Job	0.328	2.60	0.313	2.02
Full time Worker	35.858	7.33	41.386	7.82
White	11.232	2.81	11.379	2.49
Education	4.244	3.94	4.347	3.54
Worked While on Drugs	7.975	1.89	6.550	1.46
Female	–20.489	–4.43	–19.159	–3.87
Constant	–4.468	–0.32	–9.054	–0.52
Sample Size	N = 998		N = 802	

*See Table 1 for definitions of variables.
†A carat $^{(\wedge)}$ over a variable indicates that it is endogenous.

Perhaps more important, however, is our finding that drugs other than heroin lead to crime. Our results show that persons addicted to heroin gained less from criminal activities, on average, than persons addicted to other drugs of abuse. Also, the impact of drug expenditures on crime was greater for persons addicted to drugs other than heroin. Survey literature indicates that the use of drugs other

Table 4. Legal Earnings (cont'd)

| | Four Equation Model* | | | |
| | All Drugs of Addiction | | Heroin | |
Independent Variables†	Regression Coefficient	Adjusted t-Value	Regression Coefficient	Adjusted t-Value
Criminal Earnings	−0.013	−0.08	−0.123	−0.43
Sale of Drugs Earnings	−0.67	−1.36	−0.085	−1.26
Drug Expenditures	0.133	1.33	0.169	1.08
Age	−0.250	−0.37	−0.522	−0.46
Time At Longest Job	0.607	2.08	0.849	1.51
Full time Worker	42.861	5.18	46.588	4.10
White	4.518	0.61	5.095	0.52
Education	4.490	2.92	4.213	1.85
Worked While on Drugs	−3.552	−0.46	−6.042	−0.57
Female	−13.030	−2.17	−14.323	−1.60
Constant	4.179	0.20	19.61	0.47
Sample Size	N = 801		N = 653	

*See Table 1 for definitions of variables.
†A carat (^) over a variable indicates that it is endogenous.

Table 5. Drug Sale Earnings

| | Four Equation Model* | | | |
| | All Drugs of Addiction | | Heroin | |
Independent Variables†	Regression Coefficient	Adjusted t-Value	Regression Coefficient	Adjusted t-Value
Criminal Earnings	−0.766	−0.73	−0.816	−0.75
Legal Earnings	0.835	0.68	0.986	0.72
Drug Expenditures	1.632	3.53	1.497	3.55
Female	30.460	0.45	22.994	0.29
Months Before Mainlining	−0.330	−0.33	−0.801	−0.61
Heroin Addiction	−27.586	−0.34		
Constant	−6.350	−0.05	2.694	0.02
Sample Size	N = 801		N = 653	

*See Table 1 for definitions of variables.
†A carat (^) over a variable indicates that it is endogenous.

than heroin is much more widespread in the population than the use of heroin. Consequently, the greater social cost may remain with these drugs and not heroin. The potential gains to society from a more complete understanding of the drugs-crime nexus are simply too great to let the answers remain obscurred.

REFERENCES

Brown, G.F., Jr. and Silverman, L.P., "The retail price of heroin: estimation and applications," Chapter 3 of this volume.

Casey, J.J. and Preble, E. "Narcotic addiction and crime: Social costs and forced transfers." In: *Sociological Aspects of Drug Dependence,* edited by C. Winick, Cleveland: CRC Press, 1974.

DeLong, J., "Drugs of abuse and their effects." In: *Dealing with Drug Abuse,* edited by P. Wald and P. Hutt, New York: Praeger, 1972.

Drug Use in America: Problem in Perspective, 0National Commicsion on Marijuana and Drug Abuce, Second Repord, Washington, D.C.: Government Printing Office, 1973.

Ehblich, Issac, "Participation in illegitimate activities: An economic analysis." In: *Essays in the Economics of Crime and Punishment,* edited by G. Becker and W. Landes, New York: Columbia University Press, 1974.

Fuchs, V., "Male-female differentials in hourly earnings." *Monthly Labor Review,* (May 1971).

Goldman, F., "Drug markets and addict consumption behavior." In: *Drug Use and Crime,* edited by R. Shellow, National Institute on Drug Abuse, National Technical Information Service, September 1976.

Greenberg, S.W. and Adler, F., "Crime and addiction: an empirical analysis of the literature, 1920-1973." *Contemporary-Drug Problems,* (Summer 1974).

Holahan, J.F., "The economics of heroin." In *Dealing with Drug Abuse,* edited by P. Wald and P. Hutt, New York: Praeger, 1972, 255-299.

Hughes, P., Crawford, G., Barker, N., Schumann, S., and Jaffe, J. "The social structure of a heroin copping community." *American Journal of Psychiatry,* 123:5, 1971.

Juster, T.F., *Education, Income, and Human Behavior,* McGraw-Hill, 1975.

Lukoff, I., "Issues in the evaluation of heroin treatment." In: *Sociological Aspects of Drug Dependence,* edited by C. Winick, Cleveland: CRC Press, 1974.

Moore, M., "Economics of heroin distribution." In: *Policy Concerning Drug Abuse in New York State, III,* Hudson Institute, July 1972.

Patch, V., "Urban vs. suburban addict crime." In: *Proceedings of the Fifth national Conference on Methadone Treatment,* Washington, D.C.: Government Printing Office, 1973.

Silverman, L.P. and Spruill, N.L., "Urban crime and the price of heroin," *Journal of Urban Economics,* 4, 1977.

Singer, M., "The vitality of mythical numbers," *The Public Interest,* 23 (Spring 1971).

Welch, F., "Black-white differences in returns to schooling," *American Economic Review,* December 1973.

Wurmser, L., "Drug abuse: Nemesis of psychiatry," *The American Scholar,* (Summer 1972).

CHAPTER 5

Drug Addiction: Some Evidence on Prevention and Deterrence

IRVING LEVESON

The use of narcotics, marijuana, hallucinogens, stimulants, and depressants has become a major cause of concern in our society. However, until recently, drug use does not appear to have been very extensive and seems to have been concentrated among the poor in a few large cities (for data on Chicago, see Abrams et al., 1968; and Wilson, 1966). In the last few years, drug use has spread across the nation, reaching middle-class youth and suburban populations and greatly affecting the high schools and colleges. It has become a leading symptom of the "generation gap." With this growth, there has been increasing attention to the physical and mental health implications of drug use and fear that use of some of the less-dangerous drugs will be followed by growth in use of heroin and other drugs. Of particular concern has been the advent of many newer drugs which threaten to lead to a society dependent upon them, and the association of drugs with cultures which challenge the established social order (see Yolles, 1970).

The question of social policy toward drugs is immensely complex. If drug use reflects deeper problems in society—such as unequal opportunity and alienation of the young—it may be preferable to deal with those problems directly.[1] If illegal

---

[1] These may be part of the same phenomenon if the generation gap is produced by society acting as if there is discrimination by age operating similarly to discrimination by race.

drug use results in crime, one may wish to move toward greater legalization.

The issue of legalization depends upon how much it would reduce crime per addict and the way this balances against the effectiveness of penalties in curbing the size of the addict population.[2] Part of the effect of legality may depend on the way people respond to whether an act is considered legal, without regard to penalty. Much of it will depend directly upon the penalties imposed. We can obtain some very important insights into the efficacy of legalization by examining the responsiveness of the number of addicts to law enforcement activities.

There are many reasons why society may wish to reduce the number of drug addicts. Even if drug use were legal, many factors would produce external costs, such as contagion and public nuisances, which must be reckoned with. Furthermore, given the existence of a system which provides public contributions toward income maintenance, medical care, and the like, since many drug users will claim benefits, there are sizable costs to the rest of society of addiction. If we take as a constraint the existence of laws against drug possession, reductions in the social costs of crime must be counted as a benefit of efforts which reduce the number of addicts. Finally, it may not be valid to assume that drug users are fully aware of the personal consequences of their acts.

The present effort has been stimulated by observations that the effectiveness of most current drug addiction treatment programs is exceedingly low. The major exception to this is perhaps the Methadone Maintenance Program, which still deals at a treatment rather than a preventive stage, excludes most of the youngest addicts, and may not be applicable to a large proportion of the addict population (for the reasons discussed in Chapter 9). Furthermore, the criminal justice system has not produced any confidence in its ability to deal with the criminal-addict, those persons whose drug use is an adjunct of a high-crime lifestyle (as distinguished from the addict-criminal who steals to support his habit). Before billions of dollars were infused into expensive treatment systems, it was hoped that a preventive approach might be found which was more effective. In particular, it seemed important to know whether addiction might be reduced by efforts which simultaneously ameliorate poverty or improve opportunity.

This study makes some first efforts at determination of the factors influencing the number of drug users through the use of formal quantitative techniques. The purpose of the analysis is to explain changes in the use of "hard" drugs over time and to obtain evidence on the efficacy of various policy responses. We begin by examining the size and composition of the addict population in New York City and the extent to which it has grown in recent years. A wealth of data makes it possible to explore measurement problems, identify the magnitude of the drug

---

[2]The term addiction is employed in the common usage to imply drug use and not to necessarily imply either physiological or psychological parameters.

problem and the way it has changed, and obtain clues to the causes of change. The primary analysis consists of multivariate estimation of an interstate demand model of opiate use rates in 1961, in which a number of prominent hypotheses are explored. In a subsequent analysis, the effect of addiction on crime is assessed. In the final section, policy alternatives suggested by the analyses are explored.

CHANGES OVER TIME IN NEW YORK CITY

Direct Measure

The main source of data on drug use in New York City is the Narcotics Register, mandated by the New York City Health Code and financed by the U.S. Public Health Service. Since 1964, it has been deriving counts of the number of drug abusers based on reports from the criminal justice system and health and social welfare agencies (for a description of the procedures used and data beyond that presented here, see Amsel et al., 1969). The register is the most complete source available, providing much useful information about the population of known addicts.

The number of drug abusers known to the Narcotics Register by the end of 1969 was 96,649.[3] Over one-third of these (36,604) were newly reported in that year. Four out of five reported narcotics users are users of heroin.

There is no way of determining the true number of abusers of nonnarcotic drugs, but it is generally believed that few become known to authorities unless they are also using narcotics.[4]

Register personnel compared the list of deaths as a consequence of narcotic addiction for 1966 and 1967 as reported by the Department of Health with the names on the register and discovered that 53 percent were known to the register.[5] A match of deaths with the register for 1963-1969 found 45 percent listed after stratification by age, sex, and race. Since this percentage is roughly constant, it

---

[3]This includes persons reported to the register between 1964 and 1968 who have since discontinued drug use.

[4]The number of nonnarcotic drug users reported to the register is far lower than the number of arrests for possession of nonnarcotic drugs. However, the arrest statistics for narcotics include persons using both heroin and other drugs.

[5]Zili Amsel was Director of the Narcotics Register Project. The undercount may be somewhat overstated by this method since the average age of persons dying from narcoticism is lower than the general population of addicts, and the undercount tends to be greater for the young. The coverage may not be higher as a result of the accumulation of more information by the register. However, the number of addicts appears to have been growing at a more rapid pace than in the past, and relatively few new addicts are known to the register.

appears valid to multiply the register count by a constant (1½-2) to get a true figure. Furthermore, the register would tend to give an accurate indication of the magnitude of percentage changes over time.

The 1969 figure implies a rate of known drug abuse of 12 per 1,000 population with the possibility of a true rate of narcotics abuse of as high as 2.5 percent of the population. Some indication of the way the figures for New York City compare with those for other major cities can be obtained from the less complete data of the Federal Bureau of Narcotics. Data for 1969, shown in Table 1, indicate rates comparable to New York only in the nearby cities of Newark and Paterson, New Jersey. The rates for other major cities in which drug abuse has been a major concern—such as Baltimore, Washington, and Chicago—are about half the New York rate.

The New York City narcotics register provides details on the characteristics of addicts. The register has reported that four-fifths of addicts are male. About one-fourth are white, one-half black, and one-fourth Puerto Rican.

Addicts tend to be young, heavily concentrated in the 20-40 age group.[6] Addiction rates of known drug abusers by demographic characteristics are

Table 1. Comparisons of Addiction in New York City and Other Cities

	Number of Active Addicts in 1969	Addiction Rates per 1,000 Population
Baltimore, Md.	1,843	2.06
Buffalo, N.Y.	771	1.68
Chicago, Ill.	5,633	1.69
Detroit, Mich.	2,587	1.73
Los Angeles, Calif.	2,164	.78
Newark, N.J.	1,506	3.98
New Orleans, La.	714	1.22
New York, N.Y.	30,119	3.88
Oakland, Calif.	329	.92
Paterson, N.J.	763	5.33
Philadelphia, Pa.	1,502	.78
St. Louis, Mo.	254	.43
San Francisco, Calif.	705	1.00
Washington, D.C.	1,635	2.19

Source: 1971 Information Please Almanac, from U.S. Bureau of Narcotics and Dangerous Drugs.

---

[6]The national Selective Service Board recently reported that "only" two percent of the draftees examined for induction were rejected for use of hard drugs. This about equals the percentage for persons of draft age known to the New York City Narcotics Register. The Selective Service data yield an underestimate of prevalence in the age groups because of the possibility of prior rejection for other reasons (see Howard, 1970).

shown on Table 2. The male rate is more than five times the female rate, and the Negro and Puerto Rican rates are more than five times the white rate. While the Negro and Puerto Rican rates are about equal for both sexes combined, a larger proportion of Puerto Rican addicts are males. The white rate drops off rapidly in the 25-34 age group, while large declines for other ethnic groups come in the 35-44 age group.

Table 2. Narcotics Abuse Rates by Sex, Ethnicity, and Age, 1970* (per 1,000)

Total†			White		7.7
Male		33.5	Negro		40.8
Female		6.4	Puerto Rican		38.7

Age	White	Negro	Puerto Rican	Total†
5–14	.7	2.0	8.0	1.3
15–24	34.3	123.1	39.5	68.8
25–34	12.9	82.4	30.4	39.9
35–44	3.2	39.8	6.2	15.2
45+	.5	5.5	.5	1.5

SOURCE: New York City Narcotics Register and U.S. Bureau of the Census.
*The Narcotics Register excludes about half of the addicts. However it also includes former addicts who have stopped using drugs or who have moved out of the City since being reported to the Register.
†Totals include other and unknown races and drug users whose age is unknown.

The number of unduplicated additions to the register and the cumulative end-of-year totals to date have been as follows:

Year	Newly Reported Narcotics Abusers	Cumulative Total of Known Narcotics Abusers[7]
Prior to 1964	9,374	9,374
1964	6,835	16,209
1965	7,635	23,844
1966	13,107	36,951
1967	14,525	51,476
1968	19,836	71,312
1969	31,770	103,084
1970	48,137	151,221

If the number of addicts in the population were constant, the number known would tend to level off as it approached the actual number. The number of newly

---

[7]These figures refer to *Narcotics Register Statistical Report, 1964-1970 Tabulations,* May 10, 1972.

discovered addicts would tend to decline. The fact that this did not occur suggests that the number of addicts in the population has been growing, although the lack of any leveling off may simply be because the number of known addicts is still far below the actual number.

Chein et al. (1964) provides the following figures on the number of newly discovered male narcotic abusers, ages 16–20, from 1949 to 1955 from the boroughs of Manhattan, Brooklyn, and the Bronx.

Year	1949	1950	1951	1952	1953	1954	1955
Number	107	461	805	546	451	580	497

It is difficult to discern a trend during the period. There is a noteworthy jump at the beginning of the Korean War, which some observers have conjectured to be associated somehow with returning servicemen from Asia. The comparable three-borough total from the register for 1967 was about double the 1955 figure (although this may have been in large part due to improved reporting). As we shall see, the data are consistent with the notion that the current growth in addiction is associated at least in timing with military involvement in Southeast Asia.

Indicators of Addiction

Several indicators of the number of addicts are available, including the number of cases of serum hepatitis, deaths from addiction, and arrests on drug charges. All of these are subject to a strong upward trend as a result of improved reporting and diagnosis, so that while all indicate a very rapid increase in the number of known addicts, the impression given may be spurious.[8]

The Bureau of Records and Statistics of the New York City Department of Health recently constructed the following series on the number of reported cases of nontransfusion serum hepatitis, primarily due to addiction:

Year	Number of Cases	Year	Number of Cases
1960	95	1966	285
1961	178	1967	400
1962	179	1968	836
1963	166	1969	1,143
1964	190	1970	1,274
1965	168	1971	1,397

---

[8]A severalfold rise was also reported for the 1960s by the British Home Office. There is no apparent relationship between those year-to-year changes and any of our measures.

Additional insights come from examination of the number of deaths attributable to addiction (ICD Code 304); (see Helpern and Rho, 1966).

The number of narcotic deaths appears to be a good indicator of the number of addicts based on cross-sectional comparisons. The correlation coefficient between the number of narcotic deaths per capita and the number of addicts known to the register per capita across the thirty health districts of the city in 1967 was .94. However, mortality may be upwardly biased as a measure of changes over time because of improved diagnosis. It may also reflect an increasing unevenness in the strength of drugs sold rather than an increase in the number of addicts.

Table 3 indicates that the number of narcotic deaths has risen rapidly in recent years. The 794 deaths in 1970 stood at more than ten times the number in 1959. The roughly equal number of white and nonwhite deaths compared with the register's one-fourth white, indicates that the white death rate is higher than the

Table 3. Deaths from Drug Addiction by Color and Sex: New York City, 1955-1970*

	White		Other		
	Male	Female	Male	Female	Total
1955	26	6	40	10	82
1956	26	4	53	26	109
1957	33	3	40	10	86
1958	30	4	31	19	84
1959	26	4	25	21	76
1960	43	6	52	25	126
1961	103	19	116	37	275
1962	102	13	100	21	236
1963	132	25	150	35	342
1964	100	19	122	24	265
1965	72	14	28	31	195
1966	105	24	100	33	262
1967	203	22	226	39	490
1968	223	34	202	60	519
1969	274	31	323	61	689
1970	321	45	359	71	794
1971	367	55	351	94	867
1972	199	36	265	82	582
1973	204	41	215	83	543
1974	296	76	232	90	694
1975	229	53	185	62	529
1976	n.a.	n.a.	n.a.	n.a.	482

SOURCE: New York City Department of Health.
*Data for 1971-1976 added subsequent to original publication.

80   LEVESON

nonwhite rate (Burnham, 1970). The growth in the number of males relative to females is consistent with comparisons of recent counts with earlier studies of addiction. There is no clear relationship in the time pattern with the pattern of unemployment rates.

The police department has collected two kinds of statistics, the number of persons arrested on drug charges and the number of persons arrested on any charge who admit to being users of drugs at the time of arrest. Both series show the great increase in recent years that would be expected from greater enforcement activity. In 1970, there were 52,000 arrests on drug charges. It has recently been suggested that a great many addicts are arrested for loitering, usually simply because they are addicts (Burnham, 1970). This practice would tend to make the arrest statistics mirror true increases.

A rapid growth in the number of addicts in the last couple of years is suggested by data changes in the age distribution of known addicts. Persons under 20 accounted for the following percentages of heroin abusers who were newly reported to the narcotics register:

Year	1964	1965	1966	1967	1968	1969[9]
Percentage	7.3	10.3	10.8	14.7	23.6	27.7

A Closer Look at the Trends

In order to determine the extent of conformity among alternative series reflecting the number of addicts, a comparison was made of year-to-year changes in the number of narcotic deaths (D_t) with changes in the number of arrests on dangerous drug charges (A_t) since 1957 in New York City. The equation of a line fitted to the scatter is

$$D_t - D_{t-1} = a + b(A_t - A_{t-1}) + u.$$

Since we are examining changes, any linear trend is removed, and we can see whether an above-average increase in arrests is associated with an above-average rise in narcotics deaths. This would be expected if growth in the number of addicts were producing increases in both deaths and arrests, while the death and arrest rates were stable.

In the earlier years, there appears to be a negative association between narcotic deaths and arrests (Figure 1). The configuration may be spurious in view of the paucity of observations. However, the data are not inconsistent with the hypothesis that an increase in arrest with a given number of addicts reduces

---

[9]All narcotics abusers.

narcotic deaths below the number that otherwise would have occurred. The arrest variable includes a number of effects. First, the larger the number of arrests, the more addicts will be incarcerated where they cannot use drugs. An increase in law enforcement will deter some stealing by raising the probability of apprehension. Furthermore, it will increase the probability of apprehension for drug distributors. This results in a higher price for the drugs, necessitating more crime to support a habit of a given size. All these factors make for a negative association between the arrest rate and the death rate.

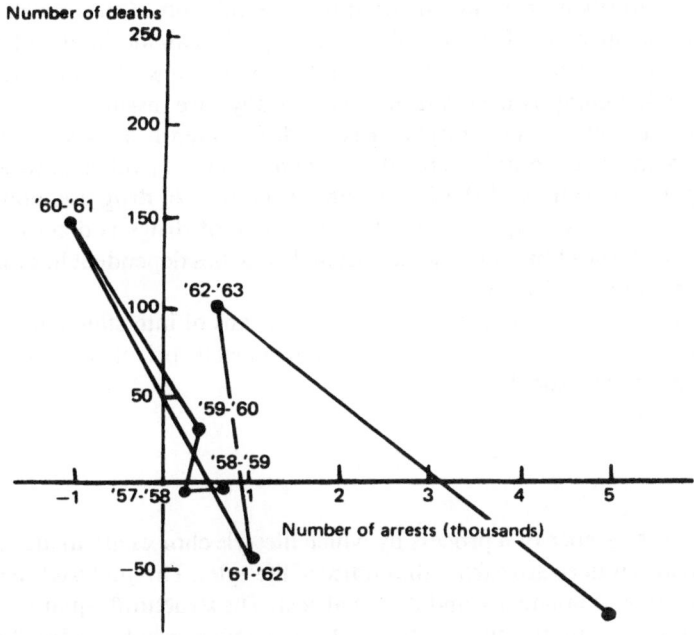

Fig. 1. Changes in Narcotic Deaths and Dangerous-Drug Arrests, New York City, 1957-1964

In the most recent years, there is no obvious relationship. Increases in drug arrests of 13,000 between 1968 and 1969 and 17,000 between 1969 and 1970 were associated with only average increases in deaths. If the death and arrests rates were constant, an increase in the number of addicts would result in a rise in the number of both deaths and arrests. This would not reduce a positive relationship which could cancel the negative tendency discussed previously. In order for this to happen now but earlier, the number of addicts would have been constant earlier and rising recently or to be increasing at a faster rate than earlier. These remarks should be taken as highly conjectural in view of the limited nature of the data, but they provide added support for the notion that there has been a real accelerated growth in the number of addicts in recent years.

THE DEMAND ANALYSIS

In spite of the rising concern for magnitude of drug use and its social consequences, relatively little is known about the determinants of the prevalence of drug use and its increase. The formulation of a model can aid in identifying critical forces. We begin by viewing the demand for hard drugs as being derived from more fundamental considerations. Specifically, we assume it to be dependent upon the choice of lifestyles. Use of drugs often is associated with irregular employment, economic dependence, and crime and other antisocial behavior. In part, the causes of the factors are also causes of drug use, and, in part, these factors are consequences of drug use. Use of drugs is determined simultaneously with the choice of other associated activities dependent in similar ways on opportunities and resources.

The determinants of drug use are examined by means of interstate comparisons in a multivariate analysis for 1961. The less technically oriented reader can skip the section on the model.

The Model

We assume the existence of a process by which lifestyle choices are made. The demand for opiates is derivative from the choice of lifestyles. The analysis focuses on the determinants of opiate use and its social cost. The structural equations of the model consist of a supply curve, a demand curve, and a social-cost function. The reduced form of the opiate supply and demand equations indicates the equilibrium number of opiate abusers. This quantity enters recurvsively into the social-cost function.

The supply curve is given by

$$D^s = \phi(P, X_1 \cdots X_m) \tag{1}$$

and the demand function is

$$D^d = \theta(P, P^d, X_{m-j} \cdots X_n) \tag{2}$$

The price of the drug is given by P, common to the supply and demand equations. An additional price P^d indicates further risks and costs to the buyer not reflected in the drug price. Both P and P^d depend on factors such as enforcement of laws against drug possession and crime generally (see Becker, 1968). P^d is treated as a shift variable in the demand function. Equating supply and demand and solving equations 1 and 2 for quantity yields the reduced form of the supply and demand equations:

$$D = f(P^d, X_1 \cdots X_n) \qquad [3]$$

The social cost function is given by

$$C = \Omega(D) \qquad [4]$$

It indicates the impact of drug use on crime, economic dependence, and the like.

The empirical analysis concentrates on the estimation of equation 2. A later section examines the impact of addiction on crime, the major component of costs to the nonaddict members of society (equation 4).

In the present model, the "price of opiates is given by exogenous locational variables representing the ease of importation. These variables are city size, which reflects the extent of international commerce and a measure of proximity to Mexico. Within the country, costs of drugs are assumed to increase with distance from these sources of supply since transportation increases the probability that penalties will be incurred. There may also be greater transaction costs in the form of penalties in dealing with smaller quantities outside the most densely populated areas. If price is exogenous, then equation 2 (the demand for opiates) is identified. Shifts in supply will tend to trace out the demand function.

Equation 2 is estimated by ordinary least-squares across 47 states in 1961.[10] The number of opiate (opium, heroin, and morphine) users per 10,000 population shown by the Federal Bureau of Narcotics in 1961 is used for the dependent variable. The regressions are run in double logarithmic form. This proved to have higher explanatory power than the linear form.

There may be a tendency for reporting to be relatively greatest where addiction is most prevalent. Also, there may be some tendency for the data to explain where addicts live rather than the "causes" of addiction to the extent migration to centers of distribution exists. This was a consideration in limiting the analysis to such large areas as states. If reporting is relatively greatest where addiction is

---

[10]The year was chosen because of the availability of several variables from the 1960 census. Data on the probability of punishment were not available for New Jersey. Alaska and Hawaii were omitted here because they have been excluded from prior studies from which most of the data were derived. The data were taken from Auster, et al. (1969), and Erlich (1970). The exchanges of data and ideas with Isaac Erlich were most valuable.

greatest, the coefficients of the independent variables will tend to be overstated, but there sizes relative to each other need not be affected. If there is migration of addicts to centers of drug distribution, we would tend to overstate the importance of supply determinants. To the extent these factors are picked up in the city-size variables, the coefficients of other variables will be more accurate.

The Variables

City Size

The strong gross association of addiction with city size may derive from a number of possible forces. If it is due to concentrations in large cities of blacks, the young, or the poor, this will be reflected in other independent variables. The city may be a more viable distribution center for drugs if concentration of addicts facilitates information transmittal or if the probability of apprehension for selling or purchasing drugs is lower when the visibility of the individual is blurred by the size of society. Urbanization may reflect tastes. The largest cities are centers for international commerce and may be easier sources of drug supply. City size is represented by two variables—the percentage of the population in SMSAs of over a million or more (SMIMM), and the percentage of the population residing in rural areas (RURAL). In view of the closeness of the association of international shipping and air transport with city size, no attempt was made to include these as separate variables.

Importation

The list of ten states with the highest opiate-use rates in 1960 includes all four of the states contiguous with Mexico, an important source of supply. Contiguity with Mexico (MEX) is represented by a dummy variable code 10 for contiguity and 1 otherwise.[11]

Punishment

The probability of punishment (PUN) measures the probability of *both* apprehension and conviction, given that an offense is committed. The measure is for all crimes. We also include a rough test of whether penalties for first offense—

---

[11]Logarithms result in a variable coded 1 and zero whose coefficient indicates its effect of the logarithm of addiction.

simple possession of marijuana—have an impact on opiate use by including a variable (MARA) coded 10 in states with a penalty of 1 year or more in prison and 1 otherwise.

Income

Income is measured by the median income of families and unrelated inviduals (MEDINC). If opiates behave as a normal good, we would expect consumption to rise with income.

Poverty and unemployment

We examine an absolute measure of poverty—the proportion of persons in families with incomes below $3,000 (ABSPOV)—and the Fuchs relative measure—the proportion of families with incomes below the state's median (RELPOV). The unemployment rate of the civilian labor force (UNEMP) is also introduced. These variables will tend to reflect lack of opportunity—i.e., opportunity costs of a life style of drug dependence. In comparing the two poverty measures, we test the hypothesis that a relative poverty measure is more meaningful than an absolute one by examining its success in "explaining" behavior.

Education

High education of persons age 25 or more (ED) would tend to be associated with high opportunity costs of addiction since the uneducated would have to forego greater earnings to participate in an addict life style. However, higher education *for a given income* would tend to be associated with lower wage rates and less employment, reflecting lower opportunity costs leaving education to be associated with less addiction. The absolute wage differential between nonwhites and whites increases with the level of education, so that for nonwhites, high education reflects lack of opportunity relative to whites even though it reflects somewhat better opportunity than less-educated nonwhites. Those with the greatest education may have a longer time preference, giving more weight to future relative to present effects. This would lead to less addiction among the more educated. If persons with a high opportunity cost of time tend to use drugs (Becker's sleeping pills) to increase the intensity with which time is used, education would tend to be associated with greater addiction (see Becker, 1965). Possible net effects include either a negative or positive partial relationship between education and addiction. In order to better understand this variable, a number of alternative specifications are examined. Separate tests were made for effects of educational levels of whites and nonwhites and variations in the proportion of the population with above and below high school education.

Demographic variables

Since young persons (YOUTH) are more likely to be addicts, the opiate-use rates should be greatest where the proportion of youths, ages 20-34, in the population is greatest. Similarly, we should find an association with the percentage of nonwhite (COLOR) if its effects are not reflected in other variables. These variables may represent either tastes or differences in opportunities.

Taste formation

It has frequently been suggested that use of drugs by youths derive from their parents' reliance on cigarettes, alcoholic beverages, tranquilizers, sleeping pills, diet pills, and excessive eating as means of responding to their problems. Usually economists are unwilling to examine taste formation, because it would be necessary to go back a step and examine the causes of parental behavior in order to arrive at an explanation of addictive tendencies. Because of this, the results are first examined without taste formation variables included. However, because of the importance of exploring intermediate points of social intervention to deal with this urgent problem, we have formulated a second model which includes taste variables. The variables tested are the annual number of cigarettes consumed per capita (CIG), the quantity of alcohol (absolute alcohol quantity) consumed (ALC), and the per capita rate of presecription drug sales (RX). In this model, coefficient of other variables reflects their impact on differences in the amount of opiate use than would be expected on the basis of knowledge of smoking, drinking, and so on. No prediction is made concerning the direction of these effects. In the taste formation model, by better controlling for other addiction variables, we would expect to obtain improved estimates of the effect of variables which influence opiate addiction but not other types of additive behavior.

The Estimates

The zero-order correlation coefficients among the variables in the analysis are presented in logarithmic form in Table 4. The strongest associations are with

Table 4. Correlation Coefficients Among Logarithms of Addiction Demand Variables Across 47 States in 1961

Variable	AD	SMIMM	RURAL	MEX	PUN	MARA	MEDINC	ABSPOV	RELPOV	UNEMP	ED	YOUTH	COLOR	ALC	CIG	RX
AD	1.00															
SMIMM	.54	1.00														
RURAL	-.61	-.49	1.00													
MEX	.35	.11	-.32	1.00												
PUN	-.31	-.30	.74	-.21	1.00											
MARA	.09	.22	.01	.06	.12	1.00										
MEDINC	.44	.38	-.69	.11	-.55	-.20	1.00									
ABSPOV	-.36	.32	.71	-.03	.56	.23	-.96	1.00								
RELPOV	-.15	-.20	.61	.08	.50	.30	-.86	.95	1.00							
UNEMP	.08	.13	.05	.08	-.02	.14	.08	-.06	-.04	1.00						
ED	.18	.07	-.46	.19	-.34	-.33	.74	-.76	-.75	-.02	1.00					
YOUTH	.19	-.03	-.25	.31	-.03	.03	.20	-.17	-.11	.02	.09	1.00				
COLOR	.38	.10	-.02	.13	.18	.36	-.38	.44	.56	.01	-.54	.34	1.00			
ALC	.40	.27	-.55	.11	-.48	-.29	.78	-.77	-.71	.13	.54	.13	-.40	1.00		
CIG	.34	.07	-.32	.04	-.22	-.17	.50	-.55	-.50	-.01	.33	.18	-.27	.72	1.00	
RX	.37	.06	-.20	.10	-.12	.14	-.13	.14	.20	-.11	-.09	.05	.43	-.13	-.18	1.00

measures of urbanization and city size. Urbanization is positively related to income and alcohol consumption and inversely related to the probability of punishment and the extent of poverty.

The measure of relative poverty clearly performs better than the absolute poverty variable. This is a significant finding since it has often been asserted that the consequences of poverty depend upon its relative effects and the relative measure appears as important for "explaining" behavior. The performance of the two measures can be seen by comparing their partial correlation coefficients. In a stepwise multiple regression, the step prior to the entry of the poverty variables is as follows:

$$AD = -3.67 + .65\,NW + 2.94\,MEDINC - 1.08\,RURAL$$
$$\quad\quad\quad (.15)\quad (.15)\quad\quad (1.14)\quad\quad\quad\quad (.54)$$

The multiple correlation coefficient is .76. The coefficients of the independent variables are elasticities; they indicate the number of percentage points which opiate-use rates change for a one percent change in each independent variable. The square of a partial correlation coefficient indicates the minimum proportion of the variation in addiction not explained by any of these variables, explained by another variable if added at this point. The partial correlation of relative poverty is .37, while for absolute poverty it is .17. The absolute poverty measure was, therefore, excluded from the subsequent analysis.

The preferred method of analysis is to specify a model which dictates the choice of variables. All of the variables designated by the model are entered together and the results examined. Under the best circumstances, a model will explain most of the variation in which there is interest by reference to only a handful of variables. With the lack of a well-developed theory and a history of empirical research, it becomes necessary to test the effects of a large number of variables, any of which might or might not be important. The need to examine a large number of variables quickly compounds with problems of measurement errors and errors in specifying the model and some high intercorrelations among independent variables to produce difficult problems of interpretation in an equation which includes all the variables under consideration. In order to deal with these problems, we have examined the order of entrance of the variables in a stepwise multiple regression in which variables are added successively and the results considered at each step.[12] The most statistically significant variables enter first. Many variables appear only in the last steps of the analysis, exhibiting lack

---

[12]In a model with two interdependent variables, the effect of multicollinearity is to increase the effect of specification error on the coefficient of an independent variable. With appropriate sizes of the parameters, sign reversals can occur. A step-wise equation which includes only one of two collinear independent variables can be interpreted as reduced form of a system of equations which includes an auxilliary equation specifying how the two variables are related.

of statistical significance at conventional levels and signs which are in some cases contrary to prediction. In presenting the equations, we therefore concentrate on the steps at which added variables still display statistical significance.

Table 5 shows representative estimates—the equation for the primary model at the end of the fifth step. The regression coefficients, indicating elasticities, are shown together with their standard errors. The coefficient of multiple correlation is .81. The significant variables in the analysis are urbanization, income and its distribution, and ethnicity. The opiate-use rate tends to be substantially lower in states with a large proportion of the population in rural areas and to be higher when a large proportion are in standard metropolitan statistical areas of a million or more persons. The strength of the tendency for areas with relatively more nonwhites to have high opiate-use rates is roughly consistent with the relative addiction rates of each ethnic group in Table 2. This is as would be expected if the variable were simply reflecting population mix. Relative poverty exerts a strong influence on addiction in addition to the influence of race. The most powerful variable is income. The effect of a one percent increase in median income is to raise the opiate-use rate by 4.7 percent. Such a high-income elasticity is quite disturbing since with real income per family in the economy growing at more than two percent per year, it implies a rate of growth of addiction in excess of ten percent per year or a doubling less than every seven years. This estimate will be considered once again in the taste formation model. The coefficients of the variables shown were not appreciably affected by the introduction of other variables.

Table 5. Primary Model Estimates of the Percentage Change in Opiate Use Rates Associated with a One Percent Change in Other Variables

	Estimated Coefficient	Standard Error
SMIMM	.09^a	.06
RURAL	−1.24^c	.55
MEDINC	4.70^d	1.46
RELPOV	3.61^c	1.71
COLOR	.40^c	.17

^{a}Statistically significant at the .10 level, one-tailed test.
^{b}Statistically significant at the .05 level, one-tailed test.
^{c}Statistically significant at the .025 level, one-tailed test.
^{d}Statistically significant at the .005 level, one-tailed test.

The list of variables which failed to enter significantly is also of interest. The probability of punishment and age variables entered in the sixth and seventh steps without statistical significance and with signs contrary to prediction. The unemployment rate, penalties for marijuana possession, and proximity to

Mexico entered thereafter with expected signs but without statistical significance. The last variable to enter was education, with a positive sign but a regression coefficient only three-tenths of its standard error. In one test of alternative specifications of the education variable, the nonwhite education variable entered fifth, after RURAL, NW, MEDINC, and RELPOV, with an elasticity of –.29 and a standard error of .18.

Next we examine the impact of different forces in explaining deviations in addiction rates from those which would be expected based on other addictive behavior. The relationship of addictive variables to opiate use and the differential effects of other variables are estimated in Table 6. The coefficient of multiple correlation is .87.

Table 6. Taste Formation Model Estimates of Elasticities

	Regression Coefficient	Standard Error
SMIMM	.14†	.05
RURAL	–.78	.51
MEDINC	2.74*	1.61
RELPOV	3.80†	1.50
ED	2.93	1.99
COLOR	.44†	.16
ALC	.47	.66
CIG	2.36†	1.00
RX	1.51*	.78

*Statistically significant at the .10 level, two-tailed test.
†Statistically significant at the .025 level, two-tailed test.

The first addictive variable to enter was alcohol consumption, with a coefficient more than three times its standard error when RURAL and NW were included. The coefficient of ALC falls and its standard error rises when CIG, with which it is highly correlated, enters the equation; when MEDINC enters, its coefficient falls to insignificance. Alcohol and cigarette consumption and prescription drug sales are positively associated with opiate use as anticipated. Urbanization, ethnicity, and poverty variables retain the same signs as before.[13] Education enters with a large positive elasticity, implying that it is important in explaining differences in opiate use from that which would be expected on the basis of other addictive behavior, but it is not statistically significant.

Income enters with an elasticity of 2.74 and a standard error of 1.61. We can use this estimate to develop a "corrected" income elasticity for opiates. We know from budget studies that higher-income groups tend to consume more alcohol,

---

[13]The absence of an effect of age may reflect particularly great underreporting of young addicts in the federal data.

cigarettes, and prescription drugs, but the differences for all of these combined are perhaps roughly proportional to income. If we assume that the coefficients of income of 4.7 and 2.7 in the two models give a correct indication of the relative effects of income on drug addiction and other addictive consumption, we would expect the drug abuse elasticity to be 4.7/2.7 times the income elasticity of other addictive substances derived from budget studies. This would imply that the income elasticity of opiate use is about 1.7, a number which appears to be much more reasonable as an estimate of long-run tendencies.

As before, the next two variables to enter after the step shown were YOUTH and PUN, with signs contrary to expectations.

The taste formation model provides a basis for obtaining improved estimates for variables expected to influence addiction toward drugs but not other substances, since other variables which may not be well controlled for are subsumed in ALC, CIG, and RX. The insignificance of the probability of punishment variable is particularly noteworthy in this context.

ADDICTION AND CRIME

Estimates of the amount of crime committed by addicts are frequently made based on estimates of the size of the addict's habit and the cost of drugs. Inferences are then made as to the amount an addict "must steal" in order to support his habit. For example, the former superintendent of police in Chicago estimated that the average cost of narcotics per day was $10 to $20, that the sale of stolen property yields about a one-fifth return, therefore the average addict steals $50 to $100 per day (Wilson, 1966). This would imply that the average addict steals $18,250 to $36,500 per year. Conservatively estimating the number of male noninstitutional addicts in New York City in 1967 as 50,000, the calculations would imply theft of $.9 billion to $1.8 billion in New York City as a consequence of addiction. This compares with the value of property stolen as reported to police of $2.1 billion in 1967 and a true value of perhaps twice that amount.[14] The implication is that addicts are responsible for one-quarter to one-half of all of the value of property loss through crime.

Somewhat higher estimates of the daily cost of drugs come from incarcerated addicts. The New York City Police Department (1967) has determined that admitted users of narcotics arrested during October 1966, averaged 4.1 bags of heroin per day at a cost of $18.33. The New York State Narcotics Addiction Control Commission (1969; Table 50) estimated the mean cost per day of the primary drugs used by certified admissions to the state program between April

---

[14]See the victimization surveys conducted for the President's Crime Commission by the National Opinion Research Center and by Albert J. Reiss, Jr.

1968 and March 1969 as $27.83. It may be that those with the biggest habits are more likely to be caught because of more frequent stealing and contact with pushers. However, there may also be underreporting of drug use.

There is a tendency to overestimate the typical amount of stealing unless one considers several additional factors.[15] While the assumption that 20 percent of the value of stolen goods is received from a fence is not unreasonable, some stealing involves cash from which the addict retains the full value. Much property is disposed of by the criminal himself, through door-to-door selling and even stealing to order, with a higher return being realized. Some income is derived through occasional employment, public assistance payments, and support from other family members. Much income is derived from "victimless crimes" such as transporting and selling narcotics, gambling, and procuring. Furthermore, shoplifting is excluded from the police statistics and victimization surveys and could well exceed a quarter of a billion dollars in New York City.

When one considers these factors, recent estimates that narcotic addicts are responsible for half the crimes committed in New York City do not seem reasonable (Institute of Public Administration, 1968, p. 231). While the estimates at hand are all quite crude, it appears that a more conservative range of one-eighth to one-quarter might be more appropriate. Even this involves an average value of property stolen of $10,000 to $20,000 per noninstitutionalized male addict per year.

Some estimates of crime attributed to addiction include nearly all crime committed by addicts whether committed as a result of the addiction or not. This is clearly appropriate for some purposes, such as estimating the reduction in crime when an addict is incarcerated and determining the impact of a psychotherapeutic program dealing with all antisocial tendencies. However, for purposes of determining the amount of crime avoided by preventing someone from becoming addicted or alleviating his physiological addiction, it is necessary to know how much more crime is committed by virtue of an additional person being addicted. Some addicts would be criminals whether or not they take drugs (Kavaler et al., 1968; New York, State of, 1968). The drug use may result in less theft than the full amount required to support the habit because with the change in life styles, less may be spent on other things. In any event, we would expect the incremental crime to be less than the total amount of crime committed by addicts.

In order to determine the effects of addiction on crime, we attempted to obtain estimates in an analysis which would provide standardization for all major forces which determine the amount of criminal activity. Isaac Erlich's (1970) National Bureau of Economic Research model of interstate differences in crime rates in 1960 explains about 75 percent of the variation in the prevalence of crimes of all

---

[15]I am grateful to John Surmeier of the RAND Corporation for many of these points.

types. The model includes variables such as income and its distribution, age, unemployment, education, and the extent of law enforcement. At my request, he was kind enough to add the Federal Bureau of Narcotics estimates of the number of opiate users per capita by state in 1961 to his equation. The result was an increase in the proportion of explained variation of four percentage points and a highly significant estimate of the affect of addiction on crime.[16] The effect of a one percent increase in the number of known addicts was alternatively estimated to increase the number of crimes against property by .04 and .09 percent. This implies that addiction is responsible for about 4 to 9 percent of all crime nationally. Higher concentrations of addicts in New York City would be expected to lead to a greater share of crime from addiction. The state crime and addiction data are, of course, also crude.[17] Yet the crime model results are consistent with other estimates of crime committed by addicts to support their habit.

DISCUSSION

The empirical analysis has primarily centered on heroin addiction. We know very little of the extent to which the results can be generalized to other drugs or other forms of deviant behavior. The present findings are by no means a perfect mirror of results on determinants of spatial variation in crime and delinquency. B. Fleischer (1966, 1963) has found juvenile delinquency related to both unemployment and income, while unemployment did not prove significant here. Ehrlich found the present relative poverty measure and a measure of the general level of income to be significant determinants of total crime rates and specific types. However, he also found unemployment and the probability of apprehension significantly associated with variation in crime, while we did not find these variables to have any relationship to opiate use.

We have suggested that opiate use is based on a complete choice of life styles influenced by opportunities. Yet the effect of addiction is to limit choice and modify the size of that response. If a person using addictive materials overestimates the ease with which he will be able to withdraw, his "decision" will take into account the opportunity costs during an underestimated expected duration of addiction. Hence he will underestimate the real costs of his initial

---

[16]The simple correlation coefficient was .68. The partial correlation coefficient was .39 and the t ratio 2.4. The results reported are unweighted double logarithmic, ordinary least squares estimates.

[17]If the proportion of known addicts increases faster than the proportion of known crimes as we move from low- to high-crime areas, the amount of crime committed by addicts will be underestimated.

behavior, which will show up as a lesser response to opportunities. On this basis, we would predict that addicts respond less to penalties for criminal activity than do criminals, but we would not predict a zero response. The modified response, if any, is reduced to too low a level to be detectable with the methods used. Had the effect been as strong as for crime, we expect that from crime studies it would have been identified.

While the data are limited, they have yielded some potentially important estimates of factors influencing the demand for opiate use. There are city-size and racial differences in drug use which cannot be accounted for by other forces. One possibility is that city size reflects the availability of drugs. The racial differences suggest that inequality of opportunity may play a significant role. Improving opportunity appears to be an important alternative to expensive addict treatment programs. The findings on the effect of poverty suggest this also.

However, poverty reduction does not appear to be an easy road. The evidence suggests it will be necessary to improve the relative position of the poor and not merely raise their incomes absolutely. This need not mean direct income redistribution, but rather improving, by whatever effective means are available, general conditions of the poor for which income is only a proxy variable. An association exists between use of opiate and use of other addictive substances. While this relationship may be caused by common factors, the evidence is not inconsistent with the notion that narcotics use can be curbed by changing behavior patterns with regard to alcohol, cigarettes, and non-narcotic drugs.

Of particular value is the estimation of the effects of variations in the probability of apprehension and conviction. First, it raises serious questions about the impact of efforts at enforcement. Furthermore, it does not lend support to the notion that legalization would produce a great expansion of the addict population.

The analysis has considered only general law enforcement and not enforcement specifically directed against drug suppliers or users. One would expect that these would increase with general enforcement, however. No hypothesis has been offered as to why enforcement is ineffective, but some interesting speculation is possible.

One way a rise in general enforcement could occur without a sizable impact on addiction is if corruption prevented it from being associated with an increase in enforcement against suppliers. The addictive nature of opiates would tend to result in low responses among those who are currently addicted, but a deterrent effect on potential addicts could also be expected. The exceptionally weak data on younger addicts do not permit a direct test of such a differential effect by age. Any selective effects of enforcement on suppliers or users could be tested if data on street prices of drugs were available. If enforcement were greater against suppliers in one area than another, it would tend to lead to higher street prices of drugs and higher value of property stolen per addict. Effective enforcement against users would tend to reduce the street prices of heroin. The problem of corruption can, of course, be examined with much more direct evidence.

Police have been reluctant to crack down on pushers, and one major reason is concern that the resulting increase in the price of drugs would lead to a substantial rise in crime (for a discussion of the enforcement problem, see Rottenberg, 1968). The evidence that the proportion of crime caused by addiction is much smaller than previously believed also suggests that enforcement against pushers is a more palatable alternative.

While the results indicate that programs dealing with addiction will not be the panacea for reducing crime some would hope for, some efforts to reduce addiction may still have sizable payoffs in crime reduction. Combining the estimates of the effects of addiction on crime with the estimates of the factors influencing addiction, we estimate that each *percentage point* of change in the index of relative poverty would be associated with approximately a two-*percent* change in the amount of crime through its effect on addiction. Also, each percentage point of change in the proportion of the population suffering disadvantages associated with race could potentially produce a two-percent change in crime through its effects on addiction.

We have only limited information on the actual growth of opiate use, but the evidence suggests it actually has been sizable even within cities. The implications of the present estimates for changes over time are disturbing. Simple application of the coefficients of the measures of income, urbanization, and addictive substances other than narcotics implies an enormous growth in rates of drug abuse in the population. While the interstate analysis considered supply variables, their applicability to changes over time is not known. Time-series patterns suggest that the Southeast Asian wars are a major factor in the growth of addiction in recent years.

The kinds of opportunity variables and policies considered in this study have been fairly traditional. It may be necessary to go far beyond them to understand the present growth of addiction, such as to simultaneously deal with the effects of a broad package of policies aimed at youth alienation.

In a society in which the logic of collective action is being increasingly brought into question, it becomes necessary to treat morality as a public good.

If the great majority of individuals have few personal objections to certain behavior patterns, but have serious doubts about the implications of similar behavior by others for the future of society as a whole, some moral regulation may be desirable. But such decisions should be based on much more uninhibited discussions of the issues than have historically taken place.

ACKNOWLEDGEMENTS

Some preliminary work on this study was undertaken at the RAND Corporation. The comments of Zili Amsel, Richard Auster, Ruth Fabricant, Elizabeth Durbin, Sidney Leveson, Frank Sloan, John Surmier, and Clarence Teng on various drafts are greatly appreciated. The views expressed are those of the author.

The paper was originally published in Urban Affairs Quarterly, December, 1972. The permission of the editors to reprint is appreciated.

REFERENCES

Abrams, A., Gagnon, J., and Levin, J., "Psychosocial aspects of addiction," *American Journal of Public Health* 58 (November 1968), 2142-2155.

Amsel, Z., Interview with author, March 1969.

Amsel, Z. et al., "The narcotics register: Development of a case register," presented at the *Thirty-First Annual Meeting of the Committee on Problems of Drug Dependence,* the National Academy of Sciences and National Research Council, Palo Alto, February 25, 1969.

Auster, R., Leveson, I., and Saracheck, D., "The production of health and exploratory study," *Journal of Human Resources* (Fall 1969), pp. 412–436.

Becker, G.S., "Crime and punishment: An economic approach," *Journal of Political Economy* 76 (March/April 1968), 169-217.

Becker, G.S., "A theory of the allocation of time," *Economic Journal* 75 (September 1965), 493-517.

Burnham, D., "City drug users placed at 3,000,000 in 7-year period," *New York Times* (May 1, 1972), 1.

Burnham, D., "Police get new rule on drug arrests," *New York Times* (November 2, 1970), 49.

Chein, I. et al., *The Road to H.,* New York: Basic Books, 1964.

Erlich, I., "Participation in Illegitimate Activities, an Economic Analysis," unpublished Ph.D. dissertation, Columbia University, 1970, Appendix F.

Fleischer, B., "Income and delinquency," *American Economic Review* 56 (March 1966), 118-137.

Erlich, I., "The effect of unemployment on juvenile delinquency," *Journal of Political Economy* 61 (December 1963), 543-555.

Helpern, M. and Rho, Y.M., "Deaths from narcoticism in New York City: Incidence, circumstances, and post-mortem findings," *New York State Journal of Medicine* 66 (September 15, 1966), 2391-2408.

Howard, P., "Draftees seldom addicts," *New York Post* (April 29, 1970), 12.

Institute of Public Administration, *A New Mental Hygiene Law for New York State,* New York, 1968.

Kavaler, F. et al., "A commentary and annotated bibliography on the relationship between narcotics addiction and criminality," *Municipal Reference Library Notes* 42 (April 1968), 45-63.

New York City Police Department, *Press Release 21,* March 1, 1967.

New York, State of, *Preliminary Report of the Governor's Special Committee on Offenders,* New York, 1968.

New York State Narcotics Addiction Control Commission, *Second Annual Statistical Report,* Albany, 1969.

Rottenberg, S., "The clandestine distribution of heroin, its discovery and suppression," *Journal of Political Economy* 76 (January/February 1968), 79-90.

Wilson, O.W., "Economic impact of drug abuse," *Illinois Medical Journal (October 1966), 522-523.*

Yolles, S.F., Statement on H.R. 11701 and 13743 before the Subcommittee on Public Health and Welfare of the Interstate and Foreign Commerce Committee, April, 1970.

CHAPTER 6

A Speculative Look at Patterns of Heroin Use Over Time

IRVING LEVESON

THE TIMING OF HEROIN-RELATED DEVELOPMENTS

National series show that there was a surge in the use of heroin and other drugs during the 1960s, especially in the latter part of the decade. However, some time between 1969 and 1973 and lasting through about 1974 the numbers of heroin abusers declined sharply. This is shown by a number of measures which to varying degrees reflect incidence and prevalence of drug use. Many interpretations can be offered to account for these changes; examples of such measures would include international drug enforcement efforts, local general law enforcement efforts, enforcement of local drug laws, and expansion of programs. We would like to better understand the changes which took place during 1969-1974, as one means of deriving insights into the effectiveness of these various measures.

Using a variety of indicators it is possible to piece together a crude picture of trends and fluctuations in heroin abuse. To allow for data limitations and for an important part of geographic variation, patterns are examined for the United States and for local areas at the same time. Along with national data, we will focus on New York City where heroin abuse is especially concentrated and

Table 1. Heroin Chronology

	Significant Developments	Significant Movements of Indicators
1965		
1966	Vietnam Buildup begins.[1]	Beginning of 5 years of rapid growth of narcotic-related deaths in New York City.[5]
1967	Sharp increase in Vietnam military activity.[1]	
1968		Narcotic-related deaths in New York City double in a single year.[5]
1969		Beginning of 7 year rise of narcotic-related deaths in Los Angeles.[6]
1970	Beginning of 3 years of rapid reduction in U.S. troops levels in Vietnam.	Sharp decline in incidence of heroin use in D.C. based on year of first use of persons in treatment.[7]
1971		Beginning of decline of hepatitis cases in New York City.[8]
1972	Turkish opium ban begins.[2] Beginning of 3 years of sharp increases in Federal spending for treatment programs.[3]	Sharp decline in narcotic-related deaths and hepatitis cases in New York City,[5,8] beginning of two years of decline in Washington, D.C. and beginning of decline in national deaths.[9]
1973		Sharp decline in hepatitis cases in U.S.[10] and in U.S. armed forces stationed in Europe.[11]
1974	Turkish opium ban lifted.	Reports of heroin influx in eastern cities.[4] Spurt in narcotic-related deaths in N.Y.C.[5]
1975	Growing reports of Mexican heroin inflow. Some reduction in Federal treatment expenditures.	Largest increase in narcotic-related deaths in Los Angeles.[6]

[1]Table 2.

[2]*Turkish Opium Ban Negotiations,* Hearing before the Committee on Foreign Affairs, House of Representatives, Ninety-Third Congress, Second Session, on H. Con. Res. 507, July 16, 1974, Washington: U.S. Government Printing Office, 1974.

[3]Sibyl Cline and Peter Goldberg, *Governmental Response to Drug Abuse: The 1977 Federal Budget,* Washington: Drug Abuse Council, 1976, Table 1.

[4]Michael Knight, "Influx of high quality, bargain-priced heroin's reported in Eastern cities," *New York Times,* December 15, 1974, p. 64; and Selwyn Raab, "Illegal narcotics traffic is worst here in 5 years," *New York Times,* December 8, 1975, p. 1.

[5]Leveson, Chapter 6, Table 3. Also see Robert Newman and Margot Cates, "The New York City Narcotics Register: A Case Study" *The Epidemiology of Drug Abuse,* edited by Mark Greene and Robert Dupont, *American Journal of Public Health Supplement,* 64 (December, 1974), pp. 24-28.

[6]S.M. Downing, "Los Angeles Police Department Narcotics Problem Evaluation," *Los Angeles: The Police Department* (June 15-17), 1976, p. 5.

[7]Robert Dupont and Mark Greene, "The dynamics of a heroin epidemic," *Science,* 181 (August 24, 1973), pp. 716-722.

information extensive, and on Los Angeles, where the experience appears to be indicative of the pattern of changes in much of the Southwest.

Table 1 presents a chronology of significant movements in indicators of heroin abuse between 1965 and 1976. These are compared with important developments potentially affecting the supply of heroin and the strength of demand. While there are serious limitations of data accuracy, the comparisons nevertheless make it possible to explore broadly which explanations of the trends and fluctuations in heroin abuse are most consistent with the historical experience.

Various pieces of data have suggested that international sources of supply play an important role. Isador Chein et al. (1964) found rapid growth in the number of young male narcotic abusers during the early 1950s, at the same time as the Korean War buildup. This also has been shown in a number of subsequent studies, including those in Chapters 2 and 3. Chapter 5 notes that all four states which are contiguous with Mexico were among the 10 states with the highest reported opiate use rates in 1961.

The chronology in Table 1 provides support for the view that the international availability of heroin has played a dominant role in accounting for aggregate variations in heroin abuse rates. An important part of the association is related to military activity in Southeast Asia.

Narcotic-related deaths in New York City rose somewhat from 1960 to 1963 and then declined between 1963 and 1965. After 1965 there were five years of rapid growth in which the number of deaths climbed from 185 to 867. The first year of that rise was when the sizeable buildup of military forces in Vietnam began. The timing and strength of Vietnam operations are indicated by the data on expenditures in Table 2. The greatest increase in narcotic-related deaths occurred between 1966 and 1967, from 262 to 490. 1967 was the year during which military activity first reached a high level. The greatest reductions in Vietnam troop levels came between December 31, 1968 and the end of 1972. This is the same period in which the decline in heroin use occurred according to the data on year of first use of persons in treatment programs (see Introduction and Chapter 2). However, direct measures of heroin abuse do not indicate a downturn until later. The peak year of narcotic-related deaths in New York City was 1971. The national decline in narcotic-related deaths began in 1972 and in

---

[8]New York City Department of Health.

[9]William Barton, "Narcotics-Related Deaths Decrease in 1972 from the Number of Narcotic-Related Deaths which Occurred in 1971," Washington: Special Action Office for Drug Abuse Prevention, Executive Office of the President, April 6, 1973.

[10]Lee Minichiello and Robert Retka, "Trends in intravenous drug abuse as reflected in national hepatitis reporting," *American Journal of Public Health,* 66, No. 9 (September, 1976), Figure 4.

[11]U.S. National Center for Health Statistics, "An outbreak of hepatitis among U.S. Army personnel-Germany," *Mobility and Mortality Weekly Report,* 23, No. 27 (July 6, 1974), p. 241.

hepatitis cases in 1973. This difference between measures makes interpretation particularly speculative.

Table 2. Levels and Changes in Troop Levels and Incremental Costs of Vietnam War

Year*	U.S. Troop Levels in Vietnam (thousands)	Change from Previous Year (thousands)	Incremental Cost of Vietnam War (billions of 1976 dollars)	Change From Previous Year (billions of 1976 dollars)
1965	184		.1	.0
1966	385	201	10.0	9.9
1967	486	100	29.9	19.9
1968	536	51	32.0	2.1
1969	475	-61	32.9	.9
1970	335	-141	25.4	-7.5
1971	157	-178	15.9	-9.5
1972	24	-133	9.2	-6.7
1973	**	-24	7.0†	-1.2†
1974	**	**	4.7†	-2.3†

*December of calendar year for troop levels, fiscal year for budget data.
†Estimated.
**Less than .5.
Source: U.S. Bureau of the Census, *Statistical Abstract of the United States*, Department of Public Affairs of the U.S. Department of Defense and Edward Fried, Alice Rivlin, Charles Shultze and Nancy Teeters, *Setting National Priorities, the 1974 Budget*, Washington: The Brookings Institution, 1973, Table 9-8, based on unpublished tabulations by the Department of Defense.

In order to understand the possible timing relationships it is necessary to inquire as to why heroin use in the United States might be related to military activity in Vietnam. One explanation is that because heroin is available cheaply and easily the servicemen themselves became addicted and brought their addiction back to the states. If returning servicemen "infected" the domestic population, domestic heroin abuse would be expected to be at its highest levels during periods when many servicemen were returning home. Since the typical tour of duty in Vietnam was one year this would imply peak rates from 1967 through 1971. While there were substantial drug abuse problems in the military services, analysis of a 1971 survey by Robbins et al. indicates that the great majority of servicemen break their habit shortly after returning to the United States rather than "infecting" many others (as would be necessary to explain the trends). In the first year after return, the proportion using narcotics fell from 43 percent to 10 percent and only 1 percent considered themselves still addicted at the end of the year (Robbins et al., 1971).

Data on U.S. forces stationed in Germany show a decline in hepatitis cases *within* a military population beginning in the fourth quarter of 1973, apparently about the same time as the declines occurred in the same measure in the United

States (U.S. National Center for Health Statistics, 1974). This must reflect something other than the movement of servicemen into the general population.

A hypothesis which could potentially explain these data is that the increased commerce with Southeast Asia which accompanied the military operations made possible the movement of opium and derivatives into the United States. Soldiers in Germany would then be affected by Southeast Asian activity levels at the same time as the civilian population. High levels of transportation and communications may have created opportunities for smuggling. The nature of the military activities themselves may also have facilitated movement of opiates to transoceanic transportation points. Such movement would be greatest when the levels of troop commitments were greatest, consistent with a peak around 1969. A high volume of transportation would have been necessary to accomplish the force reductions which occurred from 1968 to 1972 and the additional transportation opportunities may have shifted the peak forward somewhat.

The nature of the data make the suggested explanations of the relationship of domestic heroin abuse to Vietnam military activity necessarily somewhat conjectural. However, it is consistent with other experiences which also strongly suggest a major influence of international supplies. The Turkish Opium Ban of 1972 greatly reduced supplies of heroin to the United States. The timing is coincident with the decline in narcotic-related deaths in New York City and the nation. The ban was lifted in 1973 and the flow of drugs reportedly expanded in several eastern cities. New York City showed a sharp but temporary rise in narcotic-related deaths in 1974.

The growth of heroin from Mexico could account for the rise in narcotic-related deaths in Los Angeles over the entire period from 1969 to 1976. During that time deaths increased from 157 to 430. Mexican production was encouraged by market opportunities created by the Turkish Opium Ban. In 1975 Los Angeles had its sharpest rise in narcotic deaths, from 304 to 386.

What role did drug treatment programs have in the decline of heroin use in the 1970s? The rapid growth of Federal expenditures occurred over a 3-year period beginning in 1972. The proportions of addicts in treatment were modest, usually well under one fifth. Even allowing for multiplied effects through a contagion model it is unlikely that treatment was large enough nationally to be the principal cause of the decline, although that does not mean that treatment programs were ineffective. The expansion of treatment nationally came gradually through 1975 and to a significant extent it came after the sharp break in heroin abuse appeared.

In New York City the greatest growth in the number of addicts in treatment, from 30,000 to 55,000 came in 1972. (New York City Addiction Services Agency [1973].) By the end of that year as many as one third of heroin abusers may have been in treatment. Since the expansion came at about the same time as some of the international changes, it is difficult to use the New York City experience to sort out the contributions of each.

Dupont and Greene (1973) emphasize that the decline in heroin use in

Washington, D.C. was coincident with the expansion of treatment which began in 1970. As many as half of heroin abusers may have been in treatment by the end of 1972. The evidence of a sharp decline in the incidence of heroin abuse in Washington, D.C. in 1970 is based largely on calculations of age of first heroin use of persons in treatment. Narcotic-related deaths did not decline until 1972 and showed the greatest drop in 1973.

The timing of changes in heroin use is subject to considerable uncertainty as a result of differences in findings between current indicators and the historical experience as inferred from treatment data. How can we reconcile the timing based on persons in treatment with other measures? Why, even in Washington, D.C., did the number of narcotic-related deaths begin to decrease only in 1972 and show an even greater decline in 1973? To stimulate discussion and further analysis we will offer some conjectures.

Measures such as narcotic-related deaths and hepatitis cases reflect prevalence rather than incidence or reflect some combination of the two. Year of first use, on the other hand, is not only a clear measure of incidence but also may be a particularly early measure of behavior, reflecting use which occurs before it is of sufficient frequency, magnitude or duration to be reflected in other measures of incidence. Treatment programs tend to attract older users. If expansion of treatment resulted in a decline in the older users first, there would be a current change in prevalence. If supplies were less available, however, new users might be deterred more easily. If that were the case, the cumulative effects on prevalence might not appear until later. Under these conditions, year of first heroin use would be the preferred measure for present purposes.

The issue cannot be resolved at this time. Nevertheless, presently available data appear to indicate that the international supply hypothesis makes an important contribution to the explanation of observed changes and that, at least in the case of Washington, D.C. treatment program expansion and local enforcement may also have played a major role. Treatment program expansion in 1972 may also have been an important factor in New York City.

The peak may also be associated with broader social forces. The rate of growth of serious crimes generally slowed markedly after about 1969 (Leveson, 1976). These influences might be especially strong on very early use and be particularly reflected in year of first use.

FURTHER TESTS OF ALTERNATIVE EXPLANATIONS

The discussion until now has focused on the number of drug abusers and implicitly on the quantity of heroin. If the findings can be interpreted through a supply and demand model then we can obtain further evidence by examining prices. Economic theory postulates that the supply of a commodity will tend to

Figure 1

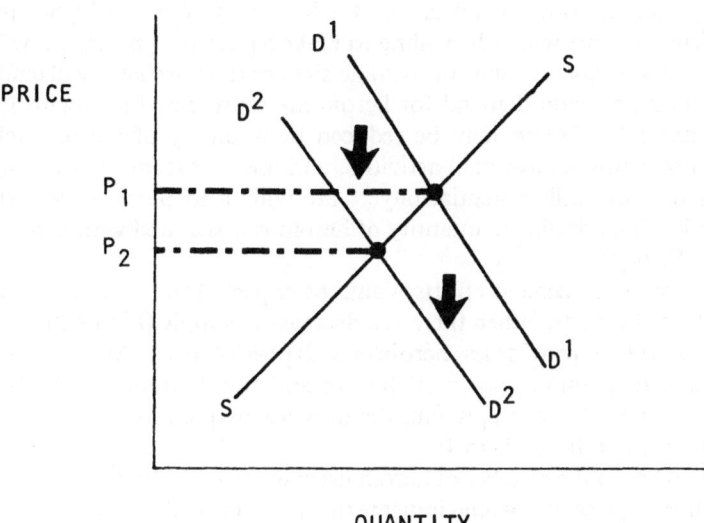

QUANTITY

Figure 2

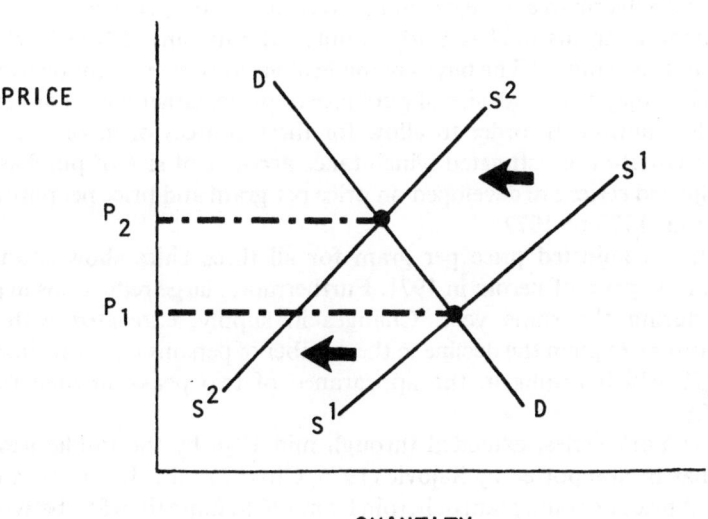

QUANTITY

be positively sloped. The least costly methods are used first and increasing prices will be required to induce production of larger quantities. The demand for a commodity, on the other hand is negatively sloped. When a higher price is charged, fewer people would be willing to make a purchase, purchases will tend to be made less frequently and the average sizes of the purchases will tend to be smaller. The supply and demand for heroin are represented in Figure 1.

The demand for heroin may be reduced by a variety of means, including treatment programs, educational activities, and law enforcement efforts against addicts. If demand falls potential buyers are willing to purchase less at each possible price. The decline in quantity of heroin is associated with a drop in its price from P_1 to P_2.

International enforcement efforts would be expected to reduce the supply of heroin to local markets. When there is a decrease in supply (Figure 2), suppliers are willing or able to provide less heroin at each possible price. Available supplies must be allocated among potential buyers and this is done on the basis of willingness to pay. When supply falls the decrease in quantity is associated with an increase in price from P_1 to P_2.

If the decrease in the number of heroin users in the early 1970s was associated with a decline in price, this would indicate that a decline in demand had occurred. If, however, the drop in quantity was associated with a rise in price it would indicate there had been a decrease in supply. (If both supply and demand are shifting the direction of price change is influenced by the shapes of the curves as well as the relative amounts of shift.) The analysis of Brown and Silverman (Chapter 3) provides the data needed for a test.

Brown and Silverman examine changes over time in the prices of "buys" made by local narcotic agents in New York County (Manhattan) of New York City, Detroit, and Los Angeles. The buys are made at various levels of the distribution system. Prices may vary with size of purchase or purity either within or between levels of distribution. In order to allow for these sources of inconsistency an adjustment equation is estimated which takes account of size of purchase and purity. Adjusted series are developed on price per gram and price per pure gram, monthly from 1970 to 1972.

The data on adjusted price per gram for all three cities show substantial increases in the price of heroin in 1971. Furthermore, large reductions in purity occurred during the same year. Changes in supply associated with these movements may explain the decline in the number of persons reporting first drug use in 1971 which results in the appearance of two peaks in Siguel's data (Chapter 2).

The New York series, extended through mid 1974 by the Public Research Institute, has been reported by Sajovic (1976, Chart 3). The data show a rise in the adjusted price per pure gram of heroin from $30 to more than $50 between the fourth quarter of 1970 and the first quarter of 1972. Between the second quarter of 1972 and the fourth quarter of 1973 the effective price surged from $48 to $108.

In the next two quarters it fell back, reaching a level of $82 in the second quarter of 1974. Data for Detroit show very similar movements, with a price change totaling 40 percent between 1970 and 1974. The most extensive change was a 70 percent decline in potency of purchases under 25 grams in October 1971. (Stoloff et al., 1975, pp. A-2 and A-3). While the data are subject to important limitations they provide further support for the hypothesis of a decline in a supply of heroin.

Evidence further suggesting that supply factors dominated the effects comes from data on the age of narcotic-related deaths in New York City. Treatment programs typically deal with persons who have been using heroin for 5 or 10 years. The vast majority of these persons are 20 years old or older. First use, on the other hand, typically starts before age 20. If a decline in the supply of heroin, reducing availability and raising the price, resulted in fewer new addicts, it would be expected to produce a sharp decline in the number of narcotic-related deaths of persons under age 20. If treatment programs produced a decline in use the effects would be expected to show up among those age 20 and over.

Table 3 reveals an interesting pattern. In the period after 1970, the decline in reported narcotic-related deaths was much sharper for nonwhite males under age 20 than it was for those age 20 and over. The same is true for nonwhite females. The size of changes for adult white males and females are similar to the magnitude for nonwhite males. The particularly sharp declines for nonwhite males and females under age 20 may be explained by either or both of the following hypotheses: 1) a disproportionate number of nonwhite youth are new users, and new users are most heavily influenced by changing availability of heroin: or 2) the especially low income of young nonwhites makes their heroin use respond more to a rise in price. Both of these explanations are consistent with the interpretation that the drop in heroin use in the early 1970s is largely the result of decreasing supplies.

SOCIOECONOMIC VARIABLES

Unemployment would not be expected to account for an upward trend in drug abuse since unemployment has no long term trend (after adjustment for changes in the age-sex composition of the labor force). Furthermore, in the years of high and rising heroin use, 1967-1969, the unemployment rate averaged 3.5 percent. Nationally the unemployment rate rose to a peak of 8.5 percent in 1975. During that period there was no rapid rise in drug abuse. Leveson (Chapter 5) observes no apparent relationship between unemployment and indicators of heroin abuse over time in New York City. In order to separate the effects of the various influences a demand model for opiates was estimated across states in 1961. The analysis did not reveal any effect of unemployment.

Recent studies of crime have found the clearest evidence of a relationship, not to the general unemployment rate, but rather to youth unemployment (Gillespie,

Table 3. Narcotic-Related Deaths in New York City
By Age, By Race and Sex, 1951-1975

Year	White Male Under 20	White Male 20 and Over	Nonwhite Male Under 20	Nonwhite Male 20 and Over	White Female Under 20	White Female 20 and Over	Nonwhite Female Under 20	Nonwhite Female 20 and Over
1951	1	10	8	18	-	-	-	3
1952	1	23	5	35	-	4	3	11
1953	3	19	4	36	-	3	1	9
1954	7	20	1	33	-	10	-	15
1955	4	22	-	40	-	6	1	9
1956	5	21	3	50	-	4	-	26
1957	10	23	-	40	1	2	2	8
1958	7	23	1	30	1	3	-	19
1959	1	25	1	24	1	24	2	19
1960	3	49	6	37	1	18	-	6
1961	16	87	10	106	1	12	3	34
1962	11	91	6	94	2	23	1	20
1963	20	111	14	106	1	18	1	34
1964	16	84	5	117	1	13	-	24
1965	12	60	3	75	2	22	-	31
1966	12	93	11	89	3	19	3	30
1967	30	173	35	191	3	19	2	37
1968	39	183	42	160	4	30	6	54
1969	75	198	83	240	10	21	16	45
1970	75	244	75	282	14	31	16	55
1971	72	295	75	276	12	43	15	79
1972	42	157	32	233	7	29	15	67
1973	33	171	26	189	3	38	10	73
1974	43	253	22	210	14	60	5	85
1975	18	211	7	178	9	44	7	55

Source: New York City Department of Health.

1975). In view of these findings it would not be surprising if youth unemployment exerted a significant influence on drug abuse which was not easily detected in analyses which lumped all age classes together. We can cite no studies which presently test this hypothesis. There are, however, a number of indirect pieces of evidence which point to a role of youth unemployment:

1. First heroin use typically occurs at ages when unemployment rates are very high.

2. The percentage of unemployed youth who are nonwhite is not dissimilar from the percentage of heroin abusers who are nonwhite.

3. Average age of first heroin use corresponds approximately with the age of leaving school, a time when high youth unemployment rates would make their influence felt.

4. A number of studies show that the most important factor in the rise in youth unemployment was the rise in the level and the coverage of the minimum wage. The major changes occurred in 1956 and 1962. Narcotic-related deaths in New York City show sharp temporary increases in 1956 and 1963.

Unlike adult unemployment, youth unemployment has a strong upward trend and this might account for some of the rapid rise in heroin abuse which occurred before 1965. It would have been expected to have a much smaller impact on subsequent trends, however. At this stage the influence of youth unemployment remains an untested hypothesis but, one which looks particularly promising.

The analysis of interstate differences in opiate use rates in Chapter 5 suggests that poverty and income are significantly related to drug abuse. The findings imply that poverty reduction would have an important, although not a dramatic effect on addiction. The evidence is based on the use of a relative measure of poverty—one that compares the position of the poor to other groups rather than examining their absolute level of income. A relative measure would be expected to change only slowly with rising incomes over time, varying largely from deliberate efforts to change the shape of the income distribution through taxes transfer payments. Reductions in poverty would have been expected to reduce rather than increase heroin use in the 1960s.

The strong estimated effect of the average level of income on opiate use rates across states implies that increases in real income over time would significantly raise opiate use. This may have had some impact in the 1960s when real income levels were rising especially rapidly. The long term consequences of such a trend if valid, must be of great concern.

Another variable found to be significantly related to opiate use is race. To the extent this measure reflects discrimination, declines in discrimination would have been expected to slow the rise of addiction.

If all of the racial differences in narcotics abuse reflected the effects of past or present discrimination it would be possible to estimate crudely the amount by which addiction would eventually fall if discrimination were eliminated by assuming that the black rates would become equal to the white rates. Data from the New York City Narcotics register shown in Table 2 of Chapter 5 suggest that with these assumptions overall narcotic addiction would fall by perhaps half. There appear to have been important declines in racial discrimination in recent years but the effects of a history of disadvantages will not disappear slowly.

DETERRENCE

During the period when drug abuse was growing rapidly the probability of a felon being sent to prison was declining rapidly. While this decline eventually stopped, there was no reversal nationally during the time when rapid declines in drug abuse occurred. This overall pattern may not be representative of individual cases.

The decline in the likelihood of punishment does not mean that additional resources were not being committed to local law enforcement. Added resources may have been channeled into an ineffective criminal justice system or they may have prevented greater drug use from occurring. However, except for the possibility of the Washington, D.C. experience, convincing evidence is lacking that local law enforcement was instrumental in producing the decline. Some aspects of deterrence are discussed in the Introduction to this volume.

Changes in enforcement together with changes in the age distribution of the population, youth unemployment and other forces are part of a phenomenon of rapidly growing crime rates during the time drug abuse was rising most rapidly and a slowing of crime growth when drug use was falling. There is much about the forces which shaped this period and influenced both crime and addiction which we do not understand.

REFERENCES

Chein, Isador, *The Road to H.*, New York: Basic Books, 1964.

Dupont, Robert and Greene, Mark, "The dynamics of a heroin addiction epidemic," *Science*, 181 (August 24, 1973), 716-722.

Gillespie, Robert, "Economic factors in crime and delinquency: A critical review of the empirical evidence," Final Report submitted to the National Institute of Law Enforcement and Criminal Justice, September 15, 1975.

Leveson, Irving, *The Growth of Crime, HI-2444/2, Croton-on-Hudson, New York: Hudson Institute, July 14, 1976.*

New York City Addiction Services Agency, Comprehensive Plan for the Control of Drug Abuse and Addiction, New York: 1973.

Robbins, Lee, Davis, Darlene, and Nurco, David, "How permanent was Vietnam drug addiction?" In: *The Epidemiology of Drug Abuse*, edited by Mark Greene and Robert Dupont, *American Journal of Public Health Supplement*, 64 (December 1974), 38-43.

Sajovic, Majda, "Crime committed by narcotics users in Manhattan," Drug Law Evaluation Project of the Association of the Ban of the City of New York, May, 1976.

Stoloff, Peter, Levine, Daniel B., and Spruill, Nancy, "Public drug treatment and addict crime," Public Research Institute of the Center for Naval Analysis, October 1975.

U.S. National Center for Health Statistics, "An outbreak of hepatitis among U.S. Army personnel—Germany," *Morbidity and Mortality Weekly Report*, 23, No. 27 (July 6, 1974), 241.

CHAPTER 7

The Effectiveness of Legal Sanctions on Individuals Addicted to Alcohol or Drugs

JAMES E. BACHMAN
ANN D. WITTE

The proliferation of property crimes and related violent crimes, particularly in urban areas, has led to increased attention to law enforcement approaches for dealing with drug abuse and other sources of criminal behavior. Analysis of the effectiveness of law enforcement has benefited from recent contributions from the field of economics. Essentially, these contributions rely on the assumption that an individual engages in criminal activity if the expected utility from this activity exceeds the utility from alternative (legal) activities. Thus the decision to commit an offense is assumed to be a rational judgment by the potential offender—an evaluation (however subjective) of the risks, potential costs, and possible benefits of a variety of activities.

However, questions have been raised as to the applicability of this "economic model of crime" to certain types of individuals such as alcoholics and drug addicts. The central issue seems to be whether or not chronic alcohol and drug users evaluate and are deterred by the risks and severity of criminal sanctions to the same degree as nonusers. A related question which has often been raised is whether these differences, if any exist, are the same for the alcoholic and the drug addict; that is, whether one might view alcohol (in the context of the economic model) as simply a potentially dangerous drug which happens to be legal in most areas. This chapter will investigate these questions by separately estimating the parameters of the economic model of crime for persons with serious drinking problems, persons with histories of drug use, and persons with no history of either problem.

The first section briefly reviews the theoretical model and cites literature from which the model has evolved. The following sections discuss the data, the empirical model, the statistical methods used in the analysis and present the results of the analysis. The final section summarizes the results and discusses the implications of our findings for future research efforts and policy making.

THE ECONOMIC MODEL

The concept of economically motivated crime is not a new idea in criminal behavior study. Since biblical times, it has been generally accepted that a thief steals to increase his own wealth. However, only recently have economists developed a formal theoretical model to explain criminal behavior.

Gary Becker began this development when he formulated a model which saw an individual allocating his time between legal and illegal activities in such a way as to maximize his expected utility from his use of time (Becker, 1968). Although the model has been revised and extended since 1968, the underlying assumption of rational choice remains the basic ingredient.

Following the early work of Becker, there have been two basic variants of the economic model. The first, developed by Isaac Ehrlich, is essentially an extension of Becker's theory (Ehrlich, 1973). An alternative model, derived by Block, Heineke, and Lind raises several questions about the underlying assumptions of the Becker-Ehrlich model.[1]

In this paper the authors will use a model which draws heavily upon the work of Ehrlich, and Block and Heineke. Under this model, an individual will evaluate his well-being (utility) as a function of his current level of wealth and his allocation of time to the following four types of activities: (1) legal income generating activity, (2) illegal income generating activity, (3) legal consumption activity and (4) illegal consumption activity. The individual's wealth, under this model, will be determined by his initial wealth and the rates of return to legal and illegal income generating activities and the amount of time he allocates to each of the income generating activities.

---

[1]Block and Lind have recently questioned a number of Ehrlich's assumptions and comparative static results. In particular, they show that a monetary equivalent for a prison term may fail to exist (1975a). In a major attack of Ehrlich's model, Block and Heineke show that if the time allocations are explicitly introduced into the utility function no comparative static results are forthcoming under traditional preference restrictions since a change in the relative return to an activity will cause an income as well as substitution effect.

Neither legal nor illegal returns are certain and hence an individual's wealth is uncertain and based on his subjective evaluation of expected returns. Illegal returns are uncertain because an individual may be apprehended and punished for illegal activity. Hence, the return an individual expects from illegal activity will depend on his subjective evaluation of the probability of being apprehended and on the cost of punishment. Legal returns are uncertain because an individual may fail to find a job. Thus the returns an individual expects from legal activity will depend on his subjective estimate of the probability that he will be unemployed.

To summarize: under this model, an individual's expected wealth will be determined by his initial wealth and the expected returns and time allocated to legal and illegal income generating activities. In turn, these expected returns will be affected by the individual's subjective evaluation of the probability of apprehension, the cost of punishment and the unemployment rate.

This model assumes that (1) time spent in job search is legal and valued at the legal wage rate but not rewarded, (2) the subjective probabilities of arrest, conviction given arrest and restriction of freedom given conviction are determinant, (3) the cost of a fine is indicated by its amount and (4) an individual will commit an integer number of offenses O, which is monotonically related to the time allocated to illegal activities (Witte, 1976b).

THE DATA

The data used in the analysis that follows consists of a random sample of 641 men who were in prison in North Carolina in 1969 or 1971. Information on the previous criminal activities and work experience of these men was obtained from the records of the North Carolina Department of Correction. The activities of these men were then followed for an average period of 37 months and an effort was made to locate and interview as many of them as possible. Interviewers were able to locate and interview approximately 71 percent of the total sample despite the often elusive and transient nature of the sample members' lifestyles. An attempt was then made to obtain complete post-release criminal records for each of the 641 men from all places the subject was likely to have lived or been arrested. A complete description of the sample and data collection is contained in Appendix A.

THE EMPIRICAL MODEL

The equation for the total number of offenses committed, O, implied by the model presented in the first section is:

$$O = f[w°, e, r, v, p(a), p(c/a), p(j/c), c(a), F, C(j)]$$

where:

$w° =$ initial wealth (wealth at the time the time allocation decisions are made),

$e =$ the expected unemployment rate,

$r =$ the expected rate of return to legal activity,

$p(a) =$ the subjective probability of arrest given an offense,

$p(c/a) =$ the subjective probability of conviction given arrest,

$p(j/c) =$ the subjective probability of restriction of freedom given conviction,

$v =$ the expected rate of return to illegal activity,

$c(a) =$ the cost of arrest,

$F =$ the amount of fine, if fined,

$c(j) =$ the cost of restriction of freedom.

In addition to the theoretical variables in the equation above, variables measuring individual tastes are included in the empirical model. Table 1 lists the variables entering the empirical equation, the measures used for them in the analysis and the sign most commonly found for them in previous studies.

Before proceeding, we should clarify several of the empirical measures. First, the variables related to the expected probabilities and costs of various criminal justice outcomes are particularly difficult to measure. The present data set provides no way of estimating the probability of arrest since we do not observe an individual's actual criminal activity. Given the fact that 80 percent of the men in the sample were rearrested during the period their activities were followed, it would seem fair to assume that the subjective probability of arrest is very high for former prison inmates. Hence the probability of arrest may be of fairly minor importance in their time allocation decision. Given the data at hand there are two possible ways of estimating expected length of sentence, EXLOS and the probabilities of conviction given arrest, $p(c/a)$ and prison given conviction, $p(j/c)$. First, we can estimate them from the past records of the individual. This would assume that individuals leaving prison form their expectations by evaluating their own past experience. This approach is intuitively appealing, allowing as it does for individual differences in ability and individual differences in offense mix. Second, we can estimate them from the immediate post-release experience of individuals who specialize in the same type of criminal activity as they do. The geographic concentration of the sample makes this assumption less tenuous than it appears at the first reading. Since the earlier work by Witte concentrates primarily on the former, we have elected to use the historical estimates for $p(c/a)$, $p(j/c)$ and EXLOS. Unfortunately, our data provided us with no measure of the cost of arrest, the amount of fines or the return to illegal

Table 1. Variables and Traditional Signs

Theoretical Variable	Empirical Measure	Traditional Sign
Dependent Variable		
O	ARRAT = Number of arrests per month free	
Independent Variables		
w^o	TPOWR = Accumulated work release funds (in $100) received after release	−
e	MFJAR = Number of months until first job after release	+
r	WAGEAR = Hourly wage rate after release	−
v	No measure	
p(a)	No measure	
p(c/a)	P(C/A) = Number of convictions divided by number of arrests prior to release from 1969/71 imprisonment	−
p(j/c)	P(J/C) = Number of convictions resulting in imprisonment divided by total number of convictions prior to release from 1969/71 imprisonment	−
c(a)	Directly related to taste variables	
F	No measure	
c(j)	EXLOS = Individual historical sentence length received (in months)	−
Tastes	AAR, AAR^2 = Age (in months) at release and its squared value respectively	+, − respectively
	AFA = Age (in months) at first arrest	−
	ARRBS = Number of arrest before incarceration in 1969 or 1971	+
	RACE = A dummy variable equal to 1 for nonwhites, and 0 for whites	conflicting
	SUPER = A dummy variable equal to 1 if an individual was supervised, e.g., on parole, when released, and 0 otherwise	−
	MS = A dummy variable equal to 1 if an individual was married, and 0 otherwise	−
	RULE = The number of rule violations during 1969/71 prison term	+

activity. Finally we note that we have no exact measure of the number of offenses committed. However, since the number of arrests is likely to correlate highly with the actual number of offenses, we accept this as our best available estimate. One further adjustment to the dependent variable was made, dividing the number of arrests by the number of months free during the follow-up to allow for varying lengths of time at risk among the men in our sample.

When attention is focused on frequent users of alcohol and dangerous drugs, the results implied by the economic model of crime may not be forthcoming. There are three reasons for expecting ambiguous results for these offenders. The first two apply to both drug users and alcoholics while the third applies only to the addicts. First, individuals under the influence of alcohol or drugs are probably less able to make accurate estimates of the probability of apprehension, conviction, and punishment. This essentially represents a breakdown in the fundamental assumption of rational choice underlying the model.[2] Second, the drug or alcohol consumption undoubtedly generates a tremendous amount of utility for the offender. Such a high level of gratification is likely to overwhelm the potential disutility of the expected criminal sanctions thereby reducing the offender's responsiveness to law enforcement. Third, in view of the cost of a narcotics habit, it is extremely unlikely that legal activity commonly available will provide sufficient income to encourage a deallocation of time from illegal income-generating activity. For example, Leveson cites two studies of addiction in New York which estimate mean daily drug costs as high as $18.33 and $27.83 per addict (Chapter 5). Faced with the high utility of the habit and the lack of legal sources of income sufficient to support the habit, the addicted offender is not likely to respond to increasing risks and costs of criminal penalties brought on by stricter law enforcement.

THE STATISTICAL METHOD

The dependent variable to be analyzed, ARRAT, required careful selection of statistical method. ARRAT, by definition, must be nonnegative. In addition, a substantial portion of our sample (20 percent) had no arrests during the follow-up; thus ARRAT = 0 for these subjects. This truncation, forced on the distribution of our dependent variable, prohibits the use of usual multiple regression techniques which rely on an assumption of normally distributed disturbances. However, the Tobit method of estimating regression equations developed by James Tobin (1958) and refined by Amemiya (1973) does permit the dependent variable to be limited in this fashion and will be used in the analysis below. Appendix B contains a statistical explanation of the Tobit technique.

---

[2]This breakdown, of course, is not limited to alcohol and drug users. A severely psychotic individual is likely to make the same errors in judgment.

THE EMPIRICAL RESULTS

The motivation for estimating separate equations for drug users, persons with serious drinking problems and nonusers lies in the results obtained in an analysis of the economic model of crime on the full sample. In the original specification for the aggregate sample, two additional taste variables ALCHY and JUNKY were included to measure the effects of alcohol and drug use on the level of criminal activity. The coefficients of these variables revealed higher arrest rates among individuals with histories of serious drinking problems or drug use, although only the coefficient of JUNKY proved statistically significant.[3]

These findings and the theoretical considerations mentioned earlier led to the hypothesis that for alcohol and drug users, the parameters of the model might differ significantly from those of nonusers. In order to test this hypothesis, we have estimated three separate models, one on a sample of 166 men with histories of serious drinking problems, one on a sample of 21 men with histories of drug use and a third on the residual group of 177 nonusers. For simplicity, we will refer to the first two groups as "alcoholics" and "addicts" respectively, although we caution the reader that such terminology should not be interpreted literally for many members of these samples.

Table 2 presents the regression equations when the independent variables consist only of the measures of initial wealth, the probabilities and costs of criminal penalties, and legal alternatives. Table 3 presents the results when taste variables are also included. An additional variable MSTAY, equal to 1 if the individual retained his work-release job after release and 0 otherwise was added to adjust for the unusually low wage rate of work-release jobs.[4]

The results of all regressions except that for the nonuser group with taste variables excluded are significant at normal levels of statistical significance. The results for addicts should be considered only indicative due to the small sample size and our reliance on maximum likelihood estimation which has desired statistical properties only asymptotically.

In the equations in Table 2, only the three criminal justice variables $p(c/a)$, $p(j/c)$ and EXLOS are statistically significant. In the case of alcoholics and nonusers, the coefficients of these variables have the traditional signs indicating a deterrent effect of law enforcement for members of these groups. It is somewhat surprising to find significant deterrence among the alcoholics but this effect may stem from the fact that a large portion of the arrests these men receive are for

---

[3]For a discussion of these results see A.D. Witte (1976b). A coefficient was judged to be statistically significant if it had the traditional sign and a one-tail hypothesis test at the 5-percent level (α = .05) led to a rejection of the null hypothesis that the coefficient was equal to zero. This criterion is maintained in the current analysis.

[4]For a discussion of this problem see A.D. Witte (1976a).

Table 2. Empirical Results: ARRAT Regressed on Direct Theoretical Variables ("t-ratios" in parentheses)[a]

Group	Constant	p(c/a)	p(j/c)	EXLOS	WAGEAR	MSTAY	TPOWR	MFJAR	$\hat{\sigma}^2$	Likelihood Ratio Test[b]
				Independent Variables						
Alcoholics (n = 166)	.6157 (4.278)	-.1401 (-1.579)	-.2392 (-2.029)	-.0013 (-2.281)	-.0242 (-1.00)	-.0606 (-1.236)	-.0041 (-.816)	-.0063 (-.867)	.0474	319.834†
Addicts (n = 21)	-1.701 (-2.715)	.6949 (3.173)	1.5766 (2.798)	-.0046 (-2.206)	.0336 (.410)	.1572 (1.173)	.0199 (1.170)	.1979 (.594)	.0307	16.373*
Nonusers (n = 177)	.4556 (2.330)	-.2421 (-2.281)	-.0457 (-.291)	-.0008 (-1.918)	-.0184 (-1.268)	-.0993 (.145)	.0014 (-1.113)	-.0309	.0674	11.756

*Indicates significance at the .05 level.

†Indicates significance at the .01 level.

[a]The t-ratios are asymptotically N(0,1) under the null hypothesis that the coefficient is zero.

[b]This is $-2 \log(\lambda)$ where $\log(\lambda)$ is the difference between the log of the maximized value of the likelihood function with only a constant term as an independent variable in the regression under consideration. This statistic is distributed χ^2_k where k is the number of explanatory variables (excluding the constant) in the regression under consideration. The statistic tests the joint significance of the independent variables and is equivalent to the F test in least squares regression.

public drunkenness and related offenses.[5] Perhaps the extremely unpleasant experience of "drying out" in local jails encourages some of them to "legitimize" their drinking by avoiding public exposure.

The coefficients for the three enforcement variables present somewhat of a paradox for the addicts. The positive signs for the probabilities imply a rise in criminal activity with increased risk, yet the highly significant negative coefficient for EXLOS reveals a strong deterrent effect of imprisonment. There are at least two possible explanations for the unexpected positive effects of risk. First, our empirical model contains no measure of the return to illegal ctivity. A possible surrogate measure, the size of the drug habit, is probably highly correlated with our measures of risk since addicts with larger drug habits will tend to make more frequent or larger drug purchases thereby increasing their exposure to law enforcement officials and a greater likelihood of arrest and conviction. Thus our subjective probability variables may actually be measuring to some extent the illegal returns, in which case we would expect the coefficients to be positive.

Our second explanation relies on our previous assumption that the utility from drugs is very high for the addict and that a legal source of income sufficient to finance a habit may fail to exist. If these assumptions are correct, the addict will require a minimum level of illegal income to support a drug habit. If we further assume (1) on the average, the addicted offender "earns" a fixed amount for every successful crime and (2) that the proportion of crimes in which he is unsuccessful is monotonically related to the proportion of offenses for which he is apprehended, any variation in the addict's illegal income will be a function of the number of offenses he commits and the rate of success he obtains. If his relative success declines (as the probabilities increase), the addict must increase his rate of criminal activity in order to maintain a given level of illegal income.

On the other hand, the expected length of sentence should have somewhat different results. In the first place, sentencing of convicted offenders tends to be somewhat arbitrary and hence, we would not expect a correlation between EXLOS and the size of the drug habit. In the second place, a possible prison term represents the potential loss of both the utility of drugs and the illegal income removing the effect of a minimum income requirement. A prison term will also add the deterrent effect of the potential disutility of undergoing withdrawal in prison and the general unpleasant experience of incarceration. Therefore, one might expect a significant negative effect of the expected length of sentence on the level of crime.

The coefficient of WAGEAR, our measure of legal income, have the

---

[5]One individual had over 100 prior arrests for public drunkenness recorded on his FBI rapsheet.

Table 3. Empirical Results: ARRAT Regressed on All Variables ("t-ratios" in parentheses)[a]

Group	Constant	p(c/a)	p(j/c)	EXLOS	WAGEAR	MSTAY	TPOWR	MFJAR
Alcoholics	.4814	−.0042	−.1186	−.0093	−.0222	−.0190	−.0024	−.0066
(n = 166)	(2.454)	(−.054)	(−1.132)	(−1.819)	(−1.048)	(−.454)	(−.532)	(−1.103)
Addicts	.5101	.2553	.4010	−.0026	−.0087	−.1362	.0395	−.9589
(n = 21)	(.309)	(1.107)	(.775)	(−1.327)	(−.127)	(−1.151)	(2.131)	(−1.345)
Nonusers	.7450	−.2168	−.0535	−.0006	−.0366	−.0679	.0054	−.0364
(n = 177)	(2.343)	(−1.952)	(−.347)	(−1.183)	(−1.119)	(−.888)	(.556)	(−1.247)

AAR	AAR²	AFA	MS	RACE	SUPER	RULE	ARRBS	$\hat{\sigma}^2$	Likelihood Ratio Test[b]
−.0006	.12 x 10⁻⁶	.0003	−.0286	−.0592	−.0436	.0082	.0177	.010	38.236†
(−.684)	(.126)	(1.161)	(−.823)	(−1.745)	(−1,194)	(.624)	(6.154)		
−.0038	.53 x 10⁻⁵	.0015	.0020	−.0179	−.4760	.0333	−.0157	.031	79.359†
(−.469)	(.458)	(.835)	(.017)	(−.223)	(−3.650)	(.927)	(−.573)		
−.0001	−.15 x 10⁻⁵	−.0006	.0330	−.0828	−.1133	.0199	−.0025	.062	29.019*
(−.066)	(−.081)	(−1.068)	(.604)	(−1.670)	(−1.941)	(1.516)	(−.215)		

[a]See footnote a, Table 2.
[b]See footnote b, Table 2.
*Indicates significance at the .05 level.
†Indicates significance at the .01 level.

negative sign for the alcoholics and non-users and a positive sign for the addicts, but none of the coefficients are significantly different from zero. Of course, in the cases of addicts, we expected that legitimate opportunity would have no effect. Our measure of the unemployment rate, MFJAR, has the traditional positive sign only for the addicts, but again, none of the coefficients are statistically significant at any acceptable level. We also obtained mixed but insignificant results for TPOWR, our measure of initial wealth when taste variables are excluded.

In general, when taste variables are entered into the equations (see Table 3), they tend to reduce the significance of the theoretical variables as would be expected with a multicollinearity problem. The only noteworthy exception to this, the positive coefficient of TPOWR, becomes statistically significant in the case of addicts. Again, this effect is not implied by the original model. The initial wealth of accumulated work-release earnings is often quite high, averaging over

$400 for men on the program in our sample. It is not unlikely that the drug user will invest much of this instant wealth in new supplies of drugs for personal consumption, thereby exposing himself to readdiction and a greater likelihood of rearrest. This, we believe, emphasizes the importance of distinguishing between the drug consumption offenses and the crimes committed to finance them. While the momentary windfall of accumulated savings may temporarily reduce the income offenses of the drug user, it is likely to increase the number of drug offenses. Unfortunately, our data does not contain information on the nature of each arrest and we were not able to further explore this potential effect.

Returning to our original task of analyzing differences between the three groups, we recall that we found considerable variation in the signs of the coefficients of several of our theoretical variables. In order to better interpret these intergroup differences, we performed hypothesis tests on the differences between coefficients found for each variable in Table 2. These differences and t statistics are presented in Table 4. The only variable whose coefficients were found to differ significantly are the three criminal justice variables p(c/a), p(j/c) and EXLOS. In addition, all the significant differences involved comparisons with the group of addicts. In the case of the expected probabilities, p(c/a) and p(j/c), these differences were significant when comparing drug users with either the alcoholics or the nonusers. This is not surprising since the signs of the coefficients are different in each case. Only when comparing drug users with nonusers is the deterrent effect of imprisonment significantly greater for the addicts. Worth noting is the fact that we found no significant differences between the alcoholics and nonusers. Thus, while the use of alcohol may result in an increase in the level of criminal activity, we have not determined that it significantly alters the magnitude of the theoretical parameters of the overall model. On the other hand, drug use not only increases the level of criminal

Table 4. A Comparison of the Theoretical Parameters ("t-ratios" in parentheses)[a]

Comparison	p(c/a)	p(j/c)	EXLOS	WAGEAR	MSTAY	TPOWR	MFJAR
Nonusers—Alcoholics	−.1020 (−.7373)	.1935 (.9853)	.0521 (.7233)	.0058 (.1415)	−.0393 (−.4265)	.0055 (.5053)	−.0246 (−8573)
Nonusers—Addicts	−.9370 (−3.850)	−1.622 (−2.773)	.3742 (1.777)	−.0520 (−.5884)	−.2565 (−1.640)	−.0185 (−.9459)	−.2288 (−.6844)
Alcoholic—Addicts	−.8350 (−3.533)	−1.815 (−3.154)	.3221 (1.502)	−.0578 (−.6764)	−.2172 (−1.524)	−.0240 (−1.353)	−.2042 (−.6128)

[a]See footnote a, Table 2.

activity but also significantly affects the magnitude of the parameters of the model, particularly with respect to the effects of enforcement.

We did not perform similar tests on the coefficients of the taste variables. However, since the administration of paroles carries important criminal justice policy considerations we did examine the intergroup differences in the effect of SUPER, which indicates whether the man was released under supervision or not. In all cases supervision was found to decrease the likelihood of rearrest, but the strongest and most significant effect was found for the group of drug users. In fact, comparative tests showed that drug users are significantly more affected by supervision than either the alcoholics or the nonusers (t = 3.19 and 2.50, respectively) while no difference exists between the non-users and alcoholics (t = 1.01). The reason for the differences involving the addicts is not immediately obvious since we would not expect that the threat of parole revocation would affect drug addicts more than other former inmates. However, the close scrutiny of paroled offenders represents a real threat to other drug users and dealers who might otherwise attempt to reestablish contact with the released offender.

If the paroled drug user is temporarily unable (or less able) to reenter the drug community, his income requirement will be low enough to allow him to postpone other types of offenses until his supervision is terminated. If this is the case, we might expect to find that legitimate opportunity may have an improved effect, at least temporarily, in reducing the allocation of time to illegal income-generating activity. Indeed, when we look at the variable WAGEAR in Table 3 we can see that the coefficient becomes negative (but still insignificant) when SUPER is included in the specification. The effects of supervision may account for the increase in significance of TPOWR, accumulated work release earnings, since parolees will be less able to purchase new supplies of drugs than nonparolees, regardless of their ability to pay for them. If we treat supervision as a measure of the relative accessibility of the drug market, an increase in available financial resources will result in an increase in the frequency that the addict takes advantage of his contacts with drug dealers, however limited they might be. Again, we must qualify our interpretation with a reminder that our ability to determine the effects of legitimate wealth (either savings or wages) on the level of crime by addicts is limited by our inability to distinguish between drug offenses and income offenses.

SUMMARY AND CONCLUSIONS

In this chapter, we have examined the relevance of the economic model of crime for persons characterized by heavy alcohol use and drug use, by separately estimating the parameters of the model from information on three subsamples of inmates who were in prison in North Carolina in 1969 or 1971. The three subsamples consisted of (1) men with histories of serious drinking problems, (2) men with histories of drug use and (3) men with histories of neither drug use nor heavy alcohol use. In effect, we have investigated empirically whether the basic assumptions underlying the economic model of crime restrict its applicability to individuals with addictive problems. In the case of both the alcoholics and the addicts we hypothesized that (1) the effects of alcohol or drugs may inhibit their ability to evaluate the likelihood and potential costs of being apprehended and convicted and (2) the use of alcohol or drugs provides a high level of utility which overwhelms the potential disutility of criminal sanctions. In addition, for drug users, we hypothesized that a legal source of income sufficient to maintain a drug habit may fail to exist. The combined effect of these factors may diminish the effectiveness of law enforcement against addicts and alcoholics.

On the one hand, we found that heavy drinkers and nonusers behave as one would expect under the economic model for criminal justice sanctions, but not for legitimate opportunity. Both types of offenders are deterred by the risk of apprehension and the expected severity of the punishment. Neither group seemed to be significantly affected by legitimate income in the form of legal wages or the savings accumulated while in prison, or by the length of time required to find a job after release, our measure of the expected unemployment rate. We also found that none of the theoretical parameters differed significantly between these two groups.

On the other hand, the drug users were found to behave quite differently from the others. While the drug addicts apparently are deterred by the expected length of a prison sentence, an increase in the probability of conviction or imprisonment seems to cause an increase in their level of criminal activity rather than the expected decrease. We offered two possible explanations for this unexpected relationship. First, we proposed that our measures of the subjective probabilities of incurring criminal sanctions correlate highly with the size of the drug habit, which would be our most likely choice for an empirical measure of the return to illegal activity for the addicted offenders. Unfortunately our data did not provide us with a measure of illegal returns and thus our estimate of the effect of risk is biased. Secondly, the combination of the high utility of drugs and the lack of an adequate legal income source may establish a minimum illegal income requirement. If the offender's return per offense declines (as we assumed might occur with stricter enforcement), his only recourse is to increase his rate of offenses to achieve a given income level. A prison sentence, on the other hand, by removing the effects of both the utility and cost of drugs would not reflect these biases and the experience of a prison term no doubt is sufficiently unpleasant due to withdrawal to deter some drug offenders. Our results also indicate that in future research attempts to analyze the economic model of crime on individual data, it is necessary to separate drug offenders from nondrug users. Our finds also show that while legal wages do not seem to significantly affect the activities of drug addicts, large sums of accumulated savings apparently promote a renewal of criminal activity upon release, probably by enabling the offenders to purchase new supplies of drugs. This effect is most pronounced when we adjusted for the level of supervision after release. Supervision was found to have the greatest effect in reducing the arrest rate of drug users. Future examination of the relationship between crime and the length of supervision and the timing and volume of the cash flow from accumulated savings may provide valuable information for correctional officials.

REFERENCES

Amemiya, T., "Regression analysis when the dependent variable is truncated normal," *Econometrica* 41, November 1973, 997-1025.

Becker, G.S., "Crime and punishment: An economic approach," *J. Polit. Econ.* (March/April 1968) *78:* 169-217.

Block, M.K., and Heineke, J.M., "A labor theoretic analysis of the criminal choice," *Amer. Econ. Rev.* 65 (June 1975), 314-25.

Block, M.K., and Lind, R.C., (1975a) "Crime and punishment reconsidered," *J. Legal Stud.* 4 (January 1975), 241-47.

Block, M.K., and Lind, R.C., (1975b) "An economic analysis of crimes punishable by imprisonment," *J. Legal Stud.* 4 (June 1975), 479-92.

Ehrlich, I., "Participation in illegitimate activities: A theoretical and empirical investigation," *J. Polit. Econ.* (May/June 1973) 81, 521-67.

Tobin, J., "Estimation of relationships for limited dependent variables," *Econometrica* 26 (January 1958), 24-36.

Witte, A.D., *Work Release in North Carolina: An Evaluation of Its Post-Release Effects,* Chapel Hill, N.C.: Institute for Research in Social Science, 1975.

Witte, A.D., (1976a) "Earnings and jobs of ex-offenders: A case study," *Monthly Labor Review* (December 1976).

Witte, A.D., (1976b) "Testing the economic model of crime on individual data," paper presented at the Southern Economic Association Meetings (December 1976).

APPENDIX A

Detailed Description of the Data Set

The immediate reason for developing the data set used in this paper was to evaluate the prisoner work release program in North Carolina. Due to this original purpose, the sample was drawn as follows. First, the population of prison inmates in the South Piedmont in 1969 and 1971 was divided into three groups: (1) a group which participated in work release in one of these years; (2) a group which was in prison in one of these years but never participated in the work release program, and (3) a group which was in prison in one of these years but participated in work release at some other time. Group 3 was dropped from consideration and Group 1 and Group 2 were considered for sampling. Before sampling the following adjustments were made. First, members of both groups who could not be followed up were eliminated. This group consisted of men who had not been released by June, 1973, men who died in prison and men who were listed as being on escape. Next all members of the non-work release group, Group 2, who were in prison for crimes which prevented their placement on work release in the 1969-1971 period were eliminated. This group consisted of all men in prison for sex crimes and serious drug offenses. In addition, all members of the non-work release population who were convicted of the public drunk offense were eliminated as they were not in prison long enough to be processed for work release. From these adjusted groups, a random sample of 297 work releasees from Group 1 and 344 non-work releasees from Group 2, were drawn. The size of the two samples was set so that an estimate of a proportion (rate of recidivism) would not differ from the population proportion by more than 5 percent, 95 percent of the time.

Interviewing of sample members took place between the beginning of July, 1973 and the end of June, 1974. The project was able to locate and interview 71 percent of the total sample. A larger proportion of former work releasees (72 percent) than men who had not been on the work release program (69 percent) were interviewed. The project was able to obtain partial information on 15 percent of the 188 men who were not interviewed. Of men not interviewed, 25 percent were located by managed to elude us, 9 percent were located but refused to be interviewed (sometime rather violently) and 66 percent were never located. The project took some consolation on its inability to locate this last group from the fact that 23 percent of them were wanted by some law enforcement agency.

If one compares the individuals the project staff was able to interview with those it was not, one finds that the old, habitual misdemeanant offender is underrepresented in the interviewed group. Hence information obtained during the interview does not adequately weight this group of individuals.

The project made every effort to obtain complete criminal records on all members of the sample whether inteviewed or not. Each member of the sample who was located was asked the date, location, and disposition of all arrests since his release from the sentence he was serving when sampled for the project (sample sentence). He was also, in a much later portion of the questionnaire, asked to indicate all areas in which he had lived since his release from the sample sentence. The criminal record in all areas where a man claimed to have lived or to have been arrested were searched to determine the validity and completeness of the criminal histories elicited from each man. Unsurprisingly, many of the men in the sample claimed substantially fewer contacts with the criminal justice authorities than they actually had.

If the project could not locate a member of the sample after extensive search, an FBI check was run to determine if a man had any criminal record which has been reported to the FBI since his release from the sample sentence. If the FBI check indicated that a man had been involved in criminal activity, the jurisdiction of this involvement was written requesting a complete criminal record. Requests for criminal records also were sent to all locations where North Carolina Department of Correction's records indicated that a man might be living.

APPENDIX B

Consider a set of independent variables Y_t^*, $t = 1, 2,..., T$. The variable Y_t^* is assumed to be normally distributed with mean $X_t\beta$ and variance σ^2, where X_t is a row vector of explanatory variables, and β is a vector of parameters to be estimated.

We observe not Y_t^* but Y_t, defined by

$$(1) \qquad Y_t = \begin{cases} Y_t^* \text{ if } Y_t^* > 0 \\ \\ 0 \ \text{ if } Y_t^* \leqslant 0 \end{cases}$$

Letting

$$\Theta = \{t | Y_t^* > 0\}$$
$$\Theta_2 = \{t | Y_t^* \leqslant 0\}$$

the likelihood function of the sample can be written as

$$(2) \qquad L = \prod_{t \in \Theta_1} f(Y_t) \prod_{t \in \Theta_2} P(Y_t^* \leqslant 0),$$

where

$$f(Y_t) = \frac{1}{\sqrt{2\Pi}\,\sigma} exp[\frac{-1}{2\sigma^2}(Y_t - X_t\beta)^2]$$

$$P(Y_t^* \leqslant 0) = F(-X_t\beta/\sigma)$$

and where F is the cumulative distribution function of the standard normal distribution.

This likelihood function (or its logarithm) can be maximized with respect to β and σ^2, using a computer, with a numerical maximization routine. This gives us the maximum likelihood estimates. Asymptotically valid tests can be constructed using the likelihood ratio principle. Alternately, we can form the information matrix. The "t ratio," formed by dividing a parameter estimate by the square root of the appropriate diagonal element of the information matrix, converges in distribution to $N(0,1)$ under the null hypothesis that the parameter is zero.

CHAPTER 8

The Effect of a Drug Education Program Upon Student Drug Knowledge, Drug Usage, and Psychological States

GLORIA A. GRIZZLE

OVERVIEW

In Charlotte-Mecklenburg, the local program developed to cope with drug abuse has three major components: (1) reducing the propensity of individuals to become drug abusers, (2) reducing the availability of illicit drugs, and (3) rehabilitating drug abusers. Fourteen schools, designated "experimental," participated in a drug abuse prevention program conducted by the Charlotte Drug Education Center. Drug usage, drug knowledge, and the percentage of students in high-risk states believed to increase the likelihood of drug usage was measured in these schools in 1972 and again in 1974. The changes in these factors were compared with changes in 12 schools, designated "controls," that did not participate in the program.

Generally, a higher proportion of students in both the experimental and control schools in 1974 than in 1972 reported using drugs, but the experimental schools reported a lower increase than the control schools. In terms of students reporting that they had never used drugs, the experimental schools did better for all drug types except alcohol. For those reporting that they had used drugs within the past month, the experimental schools did better for all drug types except alcohol (where both experimental and control schools changed by the same amount) and hallucinogens (where the control schools did better). For frequent usage within the last month the experimental schools again did better for all drug types except hallucinogens. Experimental schools also did better with students reporting that they had access to drugs but had not used them within the last year. For students who reported using drugs but not within the last year, however, the experimental schools did worse in hallucinogens, amphetamines, barbiturates, and inhalants.

The assignment of students to schools and programs could not be randomized and other changes were occurring during the period. We looked at a number of factors that might be expected to affect drug usage. It is unlikely that any of the following factors account for the relatively better performance of the experimental schools: (1) external events affecting drug usage (such as a change in the penalty structure for possessing illicit drugs and an accelerated law enforcement effort), (2) a change in pupil assignments to schools, (3) a change in the race-grade-sex composition of the students in the experimental schools compared to the control schools, (4) the school atmosphere, (5) the existence of another drug education program operating in the same school system, (6) the point at which Charlotte-Mecklenburg was located in 1972 on the time curve showing the growth and decline of drug usage, (7) a change in the percentage of students who did not respond to the questionnaire, (8) a change in the trust level of students who did respond, and (9) measurement error resulting from invalidity or unreliability of a survey instrument.

Change in Drug Knowledge

The percentage of drug knowledge questions answered correctly changed little from 1972 to 1974 in either the experimental or control schools. The average percentage of correct answers was 39 percent. Experimental schools improved relative to control schools by 0.9 percent.

Change in Psychological States

The drug education program was designed to reduce the number of students in several psychological states believed to increase the likelihood that a person used drugs. These "high-risk" states were lack of commitment, lack of attachment to school, poor parent-child relationship, hopelessness and inability to cope, boredom, rebellion, poor self-image, and peer pressure. Changes in the percentage of experimental-school students in these states compared favorably with change for the control schools only for rebellion and poor parent-child relationship. The amount of error occurring from the way these high-risk states were measured probably makes this finding unreliable. Work now underway to refine these measures may increase their reliability.

Early Intervention

A one-semester program conducted in 1972 in junior high schools with a low prevalence of marijuana usage (4.5%) was more effective in reducing drug usage than a four-semester program conducted later in schools with a high prevalence of marijuana usage (18.1%). Intensive effort in senior high schools with a high prevalence of marijuana usage (39.8%) can be effective but requires a much greater allocation of resources than does early intervention.

WHAT CHANGES OCCURRED IN THE EXPERIMENTAL SCHOOLS COMPARED TO THE CONTROL SCHOOLS?

Two questionnaires—one administered in March of 1972 and the other administered two years later—provided the data discussed in this section. Each of these questionnaires was administered to all junior and senior high school students in the experimental and control schools who were present the day the questionnaire was scheduled and who were willing to respond to the questionnaire. For the 1972 survey, 88.1 percent of students enrolled in the experimental schools responded to the questionnaire; and 85.2 percent of students enrolled in the control schools responded. For the 1974 survey, the percentages of students responding for the experimental and control schools were 78.9 percent and 83.5 percent, respectively.

Change in Psychological States

The Drug Education Center's program aimed to reduce drug usage by reducing a student's desire to misuse drugs, not by reducing his opportunity to get drugs. It was assumed that students who were in certain psychological or sociological states had a higher risk of misusing drugs than students who were not in those states. The immediate objective of the drug education program was to move some of the students in the experimental schools out of eight high-risk states. These states were rebellion, lack of attachment to school, lack of commitment, boredom, having a poor parent-child relationship, having a poor self-image, feeling hopeless and unable to cope, and feeling pressured by their peers.

**Table 1. Change in Percentage of Students in Selected Psychological/
Sociological States, Comparing Experimental with Control Schools**

State	Year	Experimental		Control		Change
		%	Change	%	Change	Difference
Lack of commitment	1972	6.7		6.8		
			0.0		0.4	−0.4*
	1974	6.7		6.4		
Lack of school attachment	1972	6.9		7.3		
			1.2		1.7	−0.5*
	1974	5.7		5.6		
Poor parent relationship	1972	57.7		57.7		
			2.0		1.1	0.9†
	1974	55.7		56.6		
Hopelessness	1972	32.3		31.6		
			.8		1.5	−0.7*
	1974	31.5		30.1		
Boredom	1972	18.2		18.2		
			1.6		2.1	−0.5*
	1974	16.6		16.1		
Rebellion	1972	19.9		18.7		
			1.1		−0.2	1.3†
	1974	18.8		18.9		
Poor self-image	1972	23.5		23.0		
			1.9		2.0	−0.1*
	1974	21.6		21.0		
Peer pressure	1972	29.0		28.8		
			1.3		1.5	−0.2*
	1974	27.7		27.3		
Ghetto milieu	1972	1.4		1.1		
			0.7		0.5	0.2†
	1974	0.7		0.6		
Incohesive family life	1972	29.7		24.9		
			−0.8		−2.1	1.3†
	1974	30.5		27.0		
Parents abuse alcohol	1972	8.8		8.2		
			0.3		−0.1	0.4†
	1974	8.5		8.3		
Illness	1972	5.4		5.0		
			−1.3		−1.1	−0.2*
	1974	6.7		6.1		

Table 1. (Continued)

State	Year	Experimental		Control		Change
		%	Change	%	Change	Difference
Loneliness	1972	38.9		38.1		
			3.1		3.5	−0.4*
	1974	35.8		34.6		
Too much pressure	1972	30.4		31.1		
			−0.9		−0.8	−0.1*
	1974	31.3		31.9		
Physician prescribes pills	1972	9.0		8.9		
			−5.9		−6.0	0.1†
	1974	14.9		14.9		

*Students in control schools did better than students in experimental schools.
†Students in experimental schools did better than students in control schools.
Experimental Schools: N = 13,919 in 1972 and 12,284 in 1974.
Control Schools: N = 11,657 in 1972 and 11,940 in 1974.

Both the 1972 and 1974 surveys contained a battery of questions that permitted estimating the number of students who were in each of 15 hypothesized high-risk states.[1] Table 1 shows the average percentage of students who were in each of these states in 1972 and in 1974 for the 14 experimental schools and the 12 control schools. One can see from this table, for example, that there was no change in the percentage of experimental school students who lacked commitment. The percentage of control school students lacking commitment dropped from 6.8 percent to 6.4 percent, an improvement of .4 percent. The control schools did better than the experimental schools in reducing the percentage of students who lack commitment.

Students in the experimental schools showed an improvement relative to the control school in only two of the eight states. They improved by .9 percent in parent-child relationship and by 1.3 percent for rebellion. For the other six states that the drug education program sought to affect, the control school students improved over the experimental school students by an amount ranging from .1 percent to .7 percent. For the seven states that were measured but not designated as objectives of the drug education program, the experimental schools did better in four instances and the control schools did better in three instances.

[1]The method of scoring responses to the questions and assigning students to these states is described in Appendix A of the full report.

Change in Drug Knowledge

Increasing students' knowledge about drugs was another program objective. Thirteen questions were included in both questionnaires to assess drug knowledge. The average percentage of questions answered correctly by students in experimental schools rose slightly from 38.0 percent in 1972 to 39.1 percent in 1974 (see Table 2). For the control schools, the average percentage answered correctly rose from 39.3 percent to 39.5 percent. Relative to control school students, experimental school students improved by .9 percent.

Table 2. Change in Average Drug Knowledge Score, Comparing Experimental with Control Schools

	Year	Experimental		Control		Change
		%	Change	%	Change	Difference
Score	1972	38.0		39.3		
			-1.1%		-0.2%	0.9%
	1974	39.1		39.5		

It should be noted that beliefs about the role that drug knowledge plays in preventing drug abuse changed during the two years that the program was being implemented. When program objectives were first formulated in the spring of 1972, it was widely assumed that providing more information about the pharmacology and physiological effects of drugs (i.e., "teaching drugs") would make students aware of the risks involved and reduce the number of students willing to experiment with drugs. As the literature suggesting that teaching drugs *per se* might in fact be counterproductive began to mount,[2] the Drug Education Center deemphasized providing drug information and concentrated more of its energies upon humanistically oriented activities (e.g., the helping relationship and decision-making skills).

Change in Drug Usage

Although reducing students' desire to use drugs by providing drug information and moving some students out of high-risk states were immediate program objectives, these objectives were not ends in themselves. They were the means

---

[2]For example, see *National Marijuana and Drug Abuse* (1973, pp.357–358) Lewis, Gossett and Phillips (1972). Swisher and Crawford (1971), and Weaver and Tennant (1973).

Table 3. Change in Percentage of Students Reporting Access to Drugs but Not Using Them, Comparing Experimental with Control Schools

Drug	Year	Experimental		Control		Change
		%	Change	%	Change	Difference
Marijuana	1972	35.3		37.8		
			4.0		6.8	2.8
	1974	31.3		31.0		
Other Drugs	1972	33.5		36.4		
			0.3		2.4	2.1
	1974	33.2		34.0		

Table 4. Change in Percentage of Students Reporting Having Never Used Drugs, Comparing Experimental with Control Schools

Drug	Year	Experimental		Control		Change
		%	Change	%	Change	Difference
Marijuana	1972	74.7		72.5		
			15.1		15.8	.7
	1974	59.6		56.7		
Alcohol	1972	53.3		50.2		
			2.5		2.2	−.3
	1974	50.8		48.0		
Hallucinogen	1972	87.8		85.5		
			2.5		2.7	.2
	1974	85.3		82.8		
Amphetamine	1972	84.4		83.2		
			3.7		4.7	1.0
	1974	80.7		78.5		
Barbiturate	1972	87.7		86.0		
			5.2		5.8	.6
	1974	82.5		80.2		
Opiate	1972	91.9		90.7		
			0.1		0.3	.2
	1974	91.8		90.4		
Inhalant	1972	79.8		79.9		
			−1.0		1.3	2.3
	1974	80.8		78.6		

through which the program sought to prevent drug abuse. Several dimensions of the change in drug usage are summarized in Tables 3 through 7—current frequent usage, remission, never used, and available but not used.

Opportunity to get drugs is one factor that figures into whether people use drugs. Table 3 focuses upon students who said they could get drugs if they had the money and if they wanted them but had not used drugs within the last year. These students presumably had the opportunity but not the desire to use drugs. In all cases, there was a lower percentage of students who had opportunity but not desire in 1974 than in 1972. The decrease in the percentage was lower for the experimental schools than for the control schools. Relative to the control schools, the experimental schools showed an improvement of 2.8 percent for marijuana and 2.1 percent for other drugs.

Another way of looking at the effect of the drug education program is to examine the changes in the percentage of students who report never having used

Table 5. Change in Percentage of Students Reporting Current Drug Usage, Comparing Experimental with Control Schools

Drug	Year	Experimental		Control		Change
		%	Change	%	Change	Difference
Marijuana	1972	13.4		15.0		
			-10.6		-11.0	.4
	1974	24.0		26.0		
Alcohol	1972	44.5		47.6		
			-2.9		-2.9	0.0
	1974	47.4		50.5		
Hallucinogen	1972	4.4		5.7		
			-0.4		0.6	-1.0
	1974	4.8		5.1		
Amphetamine	1972	4.6		5.0		
			-0.9		-1.2	.3
	1974	5.5		6.2		
Barbiturate	1972	3.5		3.9		
			-1.6		-2.4	.8
	1974	5.1		6.3		
Opiate	1972	1.8		1.7		
			-0.1		-0.6	.5
	1974	1.9		2.3		
Inhalant	1972	4.0		3.5		
			0.0		-0.7	.7
	1974	4.0		4.2		

a given drug. Reflected in these figures would be students who had not used a drug in 1972 but who would have by 1974 had there been no drug program. Not captured in these figures are those students who had used a drug but stopped using it because of the program. In every instance but one a lower percentage of students did not use drugs in 1974 as compared to 1972. The one exception was inhalant usage in the experimental schools, where the percentage of students reporting having never used that drug type actually increased from 79.8 percent to 80.8 percent. For six of the seven drug types, experimental-school students improved relative to control school students. The size of the improvement ranged from .2 percent for hallucinogens and opiates to 2.3 percent for inhalants. For alcohol, the seventh drug type, the change favored the control schools by .3 percent.

A more direct approach in determining the effect of the drug program upon drug usage is to look at the change in the percentage of students who report that

Table 6. Change in Percentage of Students Reporting Current Frequent Drug Usage, Comparing Experimental with Control Schools

Drug	Year	Experimental		Control		Change
		%	Change	%	Change	Difference
Marijuana	1972	6.5		8.0		
			−6.5		−6.7	.2
	1974	13.0		14.7		
Alcohol	1972	8.4		8.4		
			−0.2		−1.3	1.1
	1974	8.6		9.7		
Hallucinogen	1972	1.6		2.1		
			0.0		0.2	−.2
	1974	1.6		1.9		
Amphetamine	1972	1.9		1.7		
			0.0		−0.5	.5
	1974	1.9		2.2		
Barbiturate	1972	1.3		1.3		
			−0.5		−1.1	.6
	1974	1.8		2.4		
Opiate	1972	0.7		0.7		
			0.0		−0.2	.2
	1974	0.7		0.9		
Inhalant	1972	1.2		0.9		
			0.2		0.0	.2
	1974	1.0		0.9		

Experimental Schools: N = 13,919 in 1972 and 12,284 in 1974.
Control Schools: N = 11,657 in 1972 and 11,940 in 1974.

they have used drugs within the last month. In only one instance—the percentage of control students who reported using hallucinogens during the past month—did usage actually decline. The control-school change was more favorable than the experimental-school change for hallucinogens by 1.0 percent. Current alcohol usage increased 2.9 percent for both experimental and control schools. Changes in current usage of marijuana, amphetamines, barbiturates, opiates, and inhalants favored the experimental schools (Table 5).

Current usage might include students who are experimenting with drugs but who will not continue to use them as a substitute for coping with their problems. Perhaps a more appropriate measure of drug misuse would be drug usage that is both current (occurring within the last month) and frequent. Here again, the control schools showed an absolute decrease in the percentage of students reporting hallucinogen usage and a relative improvement compared with the change reported for the experimental schools. For all other drug types, the experimental schools improved relative to the control schools. The greatest relative improvement, amounting to 1.1 percent, was for students reporting that they used alcohol daily or at least several times a week (Table 6).

One final effect of the program could have been that students already using drugs stopped using them. Table 7 shows the percentage of students who said that they had used a particular drug type in the past but that they had not used that drug within the last year. The findings for this dimension of change in drug usage do not fit the pattern set for the other dimensions. In every category, a higher percentage of students reported having stopped using drugs in 1974 than in 1972. The experimental schools improved relative to the control schools only for marijuana and opiates. The control schools did better for hallucinogens, amphetamines, barbiturates, and inhalants (Table 7).

We might expect that a drug education program would have one or more of these effects upon drug usage: (1) increase the proportion of people who never experiment with drugs, (2) decrease the proportion of people who use drugs frequently, and (3) increase the proportion of drug users who stop using drugs. Several statements about how student drug usage in the experimental schools changed when compared with that in the control schools are consistent with the data presented in Tables 3 through 7. From 1972 to 1974, the experimental schools retained a higher proportion of their students in the status of nonusers than did the control schools for all drug types except alcohol. Again with one exception (hallucinogens), the experimental schools improved relative to the control schools in both the percentage of students who reported having used drugs in the past month and the percentage who reported frequent usage within the past month. Among the largest differences favoring the experimental schools were the percentages of students who said they knew how to get drugs if they wanted them but had not used them in the past year. But, for four drug types (hallucinogens, amphetamines, barbiturates, and opiates), the change in the percentage of students who stopped using drugs was greater for control schools than experimental schools.

Table 7. Change in Percentage of Students Reporting Having Stopped Using Drugs, Comparing Experimental with Control Schools

Drug	Year	Experimental		Control		Change
		%	Change	%	Change	Difference
Marijuana	1972	2.9		3.3		
			−1.5		−1.3	−.2
	1974	4.4		4.6		
Hallucinogen	1972	1.7		2.1		
			−1.3		−1.9	.6
	1974	3.0		4.0		
Amphetamine	1972	2.4		2.9		
			−1.3		−1.6	.3
	1974	3.7		4.5		
Barbiturate	1972	1.8		1.9		
			−1.5		−1.6	.1
	1974	3.3		3.5		
Opiate	1972	0.9		1.5		
			−0.9		−0.8	−.1
	1974	1.8		2.3		
Inhalant	1972	7.6		7.7		
			−0.5		−0.7	.2
	1974	8.1		8.4		

WERE THE CHANGES REPORTED CAUSED BY THE DRUG EDUCATION CENTER'S PROGRAM?

A number of factors might have affected the prevalence of drug usage in Charlotte-Mecklenburg schools in 1972 and 1973. Among these factors are a change in the penalties for possessing some drugs, school redistricting, a change in the race-grade-sex composition of the student body, the school atmosphere, the existence of another drug education program, and the maturation of the drug usage phenomenon. Other factors might not have affected the real prevalence of drug usage but might have affected the extent to which that usage was reported. These possible influences include a change in the percentage of students who did not respond to the questionnaire, a change in the trust level of students who did respond, and measurement error resulting from invalidity or unreliability of the survey instrument. Excerpts from the analysis of these issues appear below.

Changes in Drug Laws

Two changes in the North Carolina Controlled Substances Act might have affected one's perception of the risk involved in using illicit drugs and might thereby have affected current drug usage. On April 24, 1972, amphetamines were reclassified as a schedule II drug, changing the possession of amphetamines from a misdemeanor to a felony. On January 1, 1974, the ceiling on the quantity of marijuana that could be possessed and still classified as a misdemeanor was raised from 5 grams to 28 grams (one ounce). Although fewer people might have been willing to use amphetamines and more people might have been willing to use marijuana as a result of these changes in the law, there is no reason to believe that the impact upon students in the experimental schools would have been different from the impact in the control schools.

This same logic applies to other events external to the school system. Examples of other events affecting drug usage would be the increased effort by the local police to arrest users and sellers, the opium ban in Turkey, and the stepped up enforcement effort at the national level. There is no reason to believe that these events would affect the experimental schools any differently than they would affect the control schools.

School Redistricting

The Charlotte-Mecklenburg schools were under the gun of court-ordered integration during the entire history of the Drug Education Center program. Continual changes in pupil assignment plans to maintain an acceptable racial balance in each school caused a feeling of great instability among residents whose children attended the public schools. One change in school redistricting might be reasonably expected to affect the prevalence of drug usage reported in the experimental schools compared to the control schools. By the 1973-74 academic year, one of the experimental schools, under the pupil assignment plan that existed for the 1972-73 academic year, would have become more than 50% black. After several months of controversy, the decision was made to increase the size of the student body by busing in white students. The method devised for selecting the students to be bused was to draw by lot a number of quarter grids from a predominantly white section of the city and to bus all children in the affected grades who lived on the quarter grids drawn.

It might be assumed that the anxiety evidenced by the parents affected by the redistricting would be carried into the school by the students. Further, the students' attitudes about themselves and their school might change, leading to a change in drug usage reported in the questionnaire. Two methods were used to determine whether school redistricting had affected questionnaire results.

First, we broke the total number of students who filled in the questionnaire into 236 units. Each unit consisted of all the respondents who were in a particular grade and of a particular race and sex at each school. For example, one unit might have included all black, male, ninth graders who attended school X. For each unit, the change between 1972 and 1974 in the percentage of students who reported drug usage was tabulated. Using multiple regression, we estimated what the change was expected to be, based upon the sort of drug education program it had received, its age-race-sex composition, and two characteristics of the schools. We compared the expected change to the actual change for each unit and isolated the extreme units. A unit was considered extreme if its expected percentage was much higher or lower than its actual percentage.

The only pattern of extreme differences that we could detect for this experimental school was for black males in one grade who had not attended that school the previous year (N = 18). Drug usage for this unit was higher than expected for 8 out of the 29 drug usage categories. We found similar patterns in other schools not affected by school redistricting.

Next we took the percentages for the experimental school as a whole and compared them with the average percentage for all the experimental schools. There were a total of 45 categories, including 15 psychological states, 1 drug score, and 29 types of drug usage. The change for the experimental school was better than average for 24 categories, the same for 1 category, and worse than average for 20 categories. Eighty-four percent of the deviations were within three percentage points of the average for all the experimental schools. A disproportionate number of the better-than-average deviations occurred in the psychological states and the remission categories. A disproportionate number of the worse-than-average deviations occurred in the drug usage categories. School districting probably had no substantial effect upon the change in drug usage reported for all experimental schools compared to control schools. But if there was any effect, the distribution of these deviations suggests that that effect would have been to make the change in experimental school usage look worse than it actually was. It seems unlikely that school redistricting biased the survey results in favor of the experimental schools.

School Atmosphere

In looking at the effect of drug education upon student behavior, one might ask whether there are other factors in a student's life that are a much more powerful influence upon drug-taking behavior. Did the experimental schools do better because there was something about those schools that made them less conducive to drug-taking than was the case for the control schools? We tried to get at two school charcteristics that seemed important. One characteristic is the effect that the school principal has upon teacher willingness to try new methods of communicating with students. The principal's attitude toward innovative teaching methods can set the tone for the entire school. A principal unwilling to accept the risk of trying out new approaches, we assumed, could stultify a drug education program that is based upon the humanistic approach to interpersonal relations.

To determine whether the principal's willingness to innovate had affected the change in reported drug usage at their schools, we asked a member of the school administration who knew all the principals to classify each one as being either innovative, inflexible, or neutral. We then entered these ratings as variables in the multiple regression equations formulated to account for the change in drug usage for the 236 age-grade-sex units (these units are explained in the section on school redistricting). One equation was specified to explain changes in each of the 15 psychological states, the 1-drug knowledge score, and the 29-drug usage categories. We tested the innovation and inflexibility variables to determine whether their effect was significantly different from zero. The innovation variable was statistically significant at the .95 confidence level in only 3 of the 45 equations, and the inflexibility variable was statistically significant in only 1 of the 45 equations. We do not believe that statistical significance means that innovation or inflexibility really had an effect in these 4 instances. At the .95 confidence level, we would expect to conclude that there was statistical significance when in fact no effect existed in about 4 out of 80 cases. It is possible however, that a principal's innovativeness and inflexibility does affect the change in drug usage in a school and that our rating procedure was too crude a method to capture the essence of "innovation" and "inflexibility."

WERE THE ASSUMPTIONS UPON WHICH THE PROGRAM WAS BASED CORRECT?

The most critical assumptions affecting the program's logic are (1) that there are some high-risk states that increase the likelihood that a person will use drugs and (2) that a program that reduces the number of people in the states will also reduce the drug usage rate.

The Association between Psychological States and Drug Usage

Are the psychological/sociological states that are believed to lead to drug usage in fact associated with drug usage? The data indicate that most of them are. If the way these states were measured is valid, we can say that in most instances students who are in one of these states are more likely to use drugs than students who are not. Further, these states show a higher association with the categories of frequent drug usage than with the categories that include anyone reporting having ever tried a drug. The greatest association is between the state of rebellion and opiate usage. A student classified as rebellious is 4.3 times as likely to report having tried opiates and 6.5 times as likely to report having used opiates frequently.

The logic upon which this drug education program is based is that, using rebellion and opiates as an example, the drug program could move a student out of the state of rebellion and moving a student out of the state of rebellion would lower the likelihood that he would try opiates from 14.9-3.9 percent. A good test of these assumptions would be to take a group of students who are in high-risk states and randomly assign them to two groups. One group would get the drug education program and the other would not. Pre- and posttests would be given to determine whether fewer students who moved out of the high-risk states used drugs than those who remained in high-risk states. These tests could also compare the proportion in the drug education group who moved out with the proportion in the control group who did so.

Unfortunately, our guarantee to the students that they would in no way be identified made it impossible to link an individual's 1972 responses to his 1974 responses. We had to fall back to a cruder method of linking (a) the drug education program to a reduction in the percentage of students in high-risk states and (b) the reduction in the percentage of students in high-risk states to a reduction in the drug usage rate.

The method used to link the drug education program to movement out of the high-risk states was to compare the average change of the percentage of students in those states in experimental schools with the change in control schools. As previously noted (Table 1), the experimental schools improved relative to the control schools in only two of the eight states for which improvement was expected.

In an attempt to relate a change in the percentage of students in high-risk states to a change in drug usage rates, we broke the total number of control and experimental students down into 236 units. For each race-sex-grade category, we matched 1974 survey results with 1972 survey results. We then substracted 1974 percentages for each unit from 1972 percentages and linked changes in psychological state percentages to drug usage percentages for each unit. To find out whether changes in drug usage followed changes in psychological states, we set up 29 equations that would use changes in the 15 psychological states to account for changes in drug usage.

For 21 of the 29 drug usage categories, the amount of change that the psychological states accounted for is significantly (at the .95 confidence level) greater than zero. This finding of itself would not be unusual even if there were in fact no relationship at all between changes in psychological states and changes in drug usage. With 15 independent variables, we might expect an equation to fit the data enough to be statistically significant no matter what the variables were, even if the variables used had no possible relationship to drug usage. Two observations lead us to conclude that the statistical fit of the data to the equation is not simply an artifact of the statistical method used. When the 29 drug categories are looked at in terms of drug type and level of usage, a pattern is apparent. For both current usage and current frequent usage, equations for the same three drug types did not account for enough change in drug usage to be statistically significant. These drugs were hallucinogens, amphetamines, and barbiturates. The changes in the 15 psychological states accounted for only from 6-10 percent of the total variation among the 236 units in the changes in hallucinogen, amphetamine, and barbiturate usage. For remissions, the pattern is reversed. Hallucinogens, amphetamines, and barbiturates (and also inhalants) were the drugs for which a change in the psychological states accounted for enough variation among the 236 units to be statistically significant. For the drug usage categories containing students who reported having never used a drug and being able to get drugs but not having used them during the past year, all equations were statistically significant at the .95 confidence level.

Another observation concerns the significance of changes in individual psychological states, as opposed to the significance of changes in all 15 psychological states combined. The effects of these states are greater than zero (at the .95 confidence level) too often—63 out of 435 instances—to have occurred by chance alone.

While there is reason to believe that the changes in the 15 psychological states do account for some of the variation among the 236 units in changes in drug usage, the percentage of total variation accounted for is small. The amount of variation that the change in psychological states "explains" for the 21 drug categories having statistically significant equations ranges from 13 percent up to 20 percent.

We know that there is an association between reported drug usage and these psychological states (as measured using the 1972 and 1974 questionnaires). We also know that this relationship is fairly stable over the two-year period. Given the stable association between high-risk states and drug usage, there are several possible reasons for the changes in the psychological states explaining so little of the changes in drug usage. For at least some of the psychological states, the direction of causation might be the reverse of the direction we assumed. Perhaps a poor parent-child relationship, or rebellion, or boredom, and so forth, are caused by using drugs instead of causing drug usage. Another possible reason is that there is some factor (or factors) not yet articulated that affects both the high-risk states and drug usage and that neither being in the high-risk states causes one to use drugs nor using drugs causes one to be in the high-risk states. A third possible reason is that measurement error was so great in the data used to test the logic upon which the program was based that the causal relationship was washed out.

There was little change from 1972 to 1974 in the percentage of students classified as being in the high-risk states. In attempting to account for the change in drug usage in terms of the difference between the 1972 and 1974 percentages, we are dealing with factors having a very small magnitude. For the entire student body, only two of the 15 states changed by more than 2 percent. The state showing the largest change, physician prescribing drugs, was statistically significant in 12 of the 29 equations explaining a change in drug usage in terms of a change in psychological/sociological states. The average for all the psychological/sociological states is only three equations. Thus if the change in percentages had been larger, the equations might have accounted for substantially more of the changes in drug usage. Measurement error that might be tolerable in establishing an association between a psychological state (where the percentages range up to 57 percent) and drug usage might not be tolerable in establishing an association between the change in a psychological state (where most percentages are less than 2 percent) and a change in drug usage.

HOW GENERAL AND PERMANENT ARE THE EFFECTS?

Students Most Likely to Benefit from the Drug Education Program

Did the drug education program affect attitudes and usage in some grade-race-sex groupings more than others? To answer this question, we broke the experimental and control school changes down for three psychological states and 5-drug usage categories and tabulated each instance in which a grade-race-sex category in the experimental schools did better than that same category in the control schools. No grade-sex-race combination of experimental students did either better or worse than their control school counterparts across all eight psychological and drug usage categories. We found no pattern that suggests that some grade-sex-race categories benefitted from the drug education program more than others.

Does a Reduction in Drug Use Continue After the Drug Education Program Ends?

To answer this question, we compared changes in drug usage rates for three groups of schools. The early program group consisted of those experimental schools that participated in the drug education program in the spring semester of 1972 but not in the 1972-73 and 1973-74 academic years. Note that the second survey was given almost two years after the drug education program ended in those schools. The recent program group included the schools that were in the program during the 1972-73 and 1973-74 academic years. Control schools made up the third group.

Table 8. Change in Reported Marijuana Usage by Type of Drug Education Program

	Percentage of Students Who Have Ever Used Marijuana				
Type of Drug Education Program Received	1969 Survey	1972 Survey	1974 Survey	Change 1969-1972	1972-1974
Junior High School					
Early	4.5%	12.9%	23.0%	8.4%	10.1%
Recent	7.4	18.1	32.2	10.7	14.1
None	5.8	16.1	28.9	10.3	12.8
Senior High School					
Early	8.7	28.4	47.4	19.7	19.0
Recent	15.9	39.8	58.3	23.9	18.5
None	10.5	35.1	55.5	24.6	20.4

Because we needed to look at drug usage at three points in time, we focused upon marijuana, the only drug covered individually in the survey that the Mecklenburg County Medical Society conducted in November, 1969. We would expect the early program schools to improve relative to the recent program and control schools between 1969 and 1972; likewise, we would expect the recent program schools to improve relative to the other two groups between 1972 and 1974. Senior high schools showed the expected relative improvements. From 1969 to 1972, the percentage increase in students reporting having ever used marijuana was lowest for the early program (19.7 percent compared to 23.9 percent and 24.6 percent for the other groups). From 1972 to 1974, the percentage increase was lowest for the recent program (Table 8).

Such is not the case for the junior high schools. From 1969 to 1972, the changes fit our expectations, with the early program schools having the lowest increase. But the recent program schools showed the highest increase instead of the lowest increase between 1972 and 1974. In searching for an explanation for this last finding, we divided all the junior high schools into two groups, one group having a low prevalence of reported marijuana usage in 1969 and the other having a high prevalence. All the early program schools fell into the low-prevalence group and all the recent program schools fell into the high-prevalence group.

What caused the low-prevalence experimental (early program) schools to increase drug usage at a lower rate between 1972 and 1974 than the high-prevalence experimental (recent program) schools? Would the rate of increase

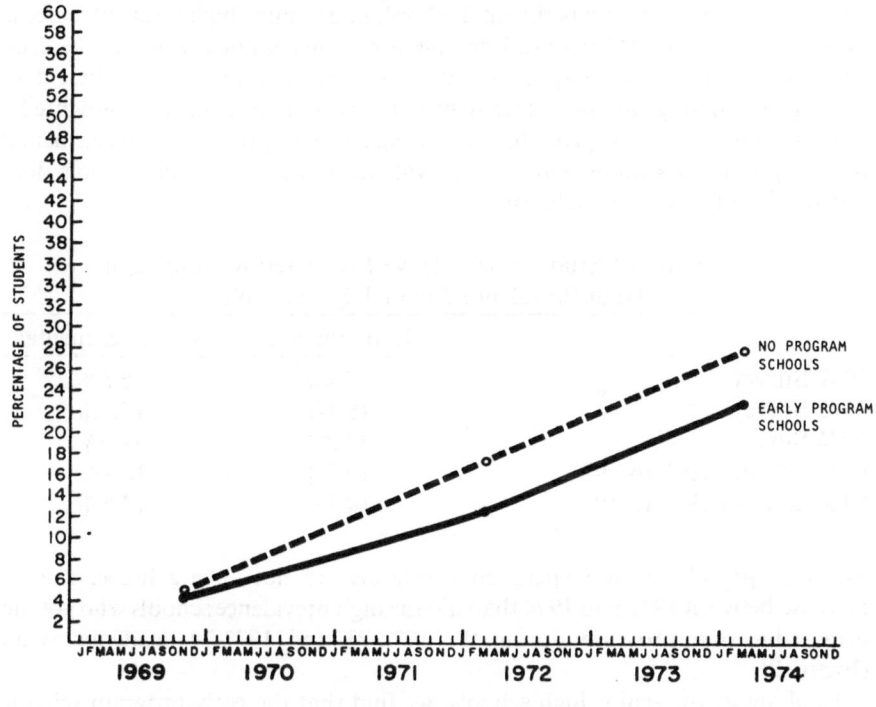

Fig. 1. Change in Percentage of Junior High School Students Reporting Having Ever Used Marijuana, Low Prevalence Schools.

for the low-prevalence experimental schools have been lower without the program simply because drug usage rises slowest in schools with the lowest prevalence? We compared the low-prevalence experimental schools with the low-prevalence nonexperimental schools:

Percentage of Students Who Have Ever Used Marijuana in Low Prevalence Junior High Schools

	Experimental	Nonexperimental
1969 Survey	4.5%	4.8%
1972 Survey	12.9%	17.6%
1974 Survey	23.0%	28.1%
Change from 1969 to 1972	8.4%	12.8%
Change from 1972 to 1974	10.1%	10.5%

The low-prevalence nonexperimental schools had a much higher rate of increase between 1969 and 1972 than did the low-prevalence schools who got the drug education program in the spring of 1972. One might conclude from these data that the recent program did indeed reduce the rate of marijuana usage (Figure 1).

Following a similar procedure to compare high-prevalence experimental (recent program) schools with high-prevalence nonexperimental schools does not result in a similar conclusion.

Percentage of Students who Have Ever Used Marijuana in
High-Prevalence Junior High Schools

	Experimental	Nonexperimental
1969 Survey	7.4%	6.8%
1972 Survey	18.1%	17.7%
1974 Survey	32.2%	31.2%
Change from 1969 to 1972	10.7%	10.9%
Change from 1972 to 1974	14.1%	13.5%

The high-prevalence nonexperimental schools did not have a higher rate of increase between 1972 and 1974 than did the high prevalence schools who got the drug education program during the 1972-73 and 1973-74 academic years (Figure 2).

Looking at the senior high schools, we find that the early program schools were low-prevalence schools in 1969 and that the recent programs were high-prevalence schools. Yet the high-prevalence recent program schools still did better than the control schools between 1972 and 1974. The apparent reason is that the two senior high schools during 1973-74 were given a much more intensive program than the six junior high schools received.

What do these different rates of change say to us about drug education programs? This interpretation is consistent with the data: A program designed to prevent experimental usage of drugs will be much more effective if the program is implemented when the prevalence of experimental usage is low (around 4 or 5 percent). If program intervention does not come until the prevalence of experimental usage has reached about 15 percent, it can still prevent experimental usage. But to do so, the resources invested must be much greater (about tenfold) to achieve the results than could be obtained from early intervention. This attribution of reduced drug usage to early intervention could be incorrect if there were other conditions that affected the low-prevalence early program schools but not the low prevalence of nonexperimental schools. We do not know that there were any such conditions but we do not have the information needed to rule out that possibility.

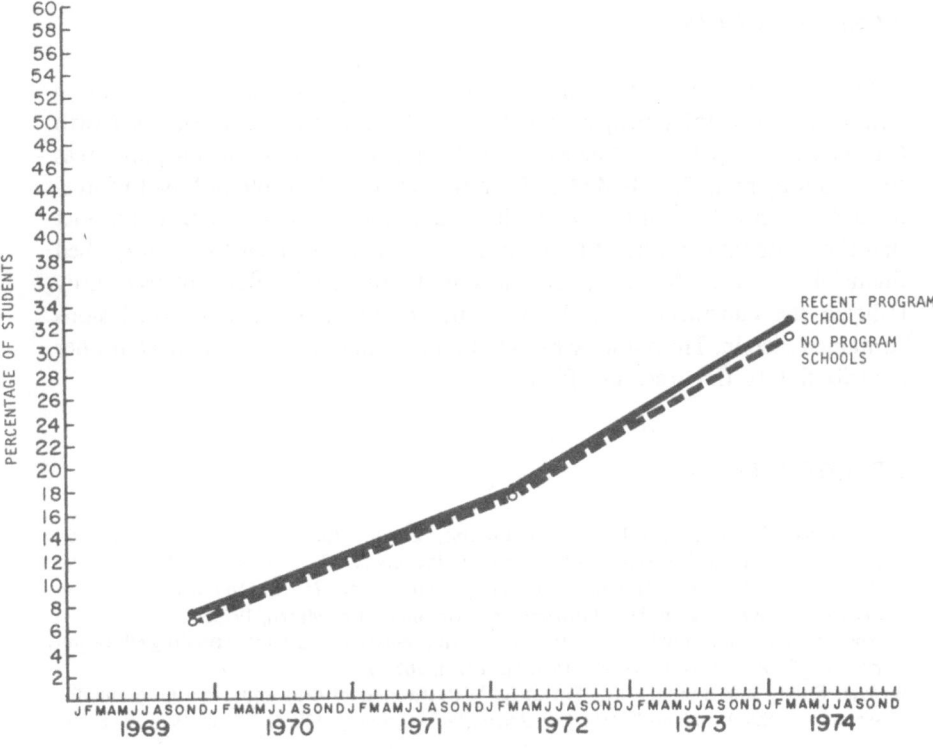

Fig. 2. Change In Percentage Of Junior High School Students Reporting Having Ever Used Marijuana. High-Prevalence Schools.

Length of Program Exposure

Students who attended for a two-year period one of the schools that had the recent drug program showed more favorable change in both the psychological states and drug usage categories than students who attended one of these schools only in 1973-74. We included length of program exposure as an independent variable along with variables defining the drug education program the school received, the innovativeness or inflexibility of the principal, school size, grade, race, and sex. At the .95 confidence level, length of program exposure accounted for enough change to be statistically significant in 6 of the 15 psychological states and 8 of the 29 drug usage categories. Statistical significance occurs too frequently to attribute these results to chance variation.

ACKNOWLEDGMENTS

This paper is excerpted from a report by the same title of the Mecklenburg Criminal Justice Pilot Project, Institute of Government, University of North Carolina at Chapel Hill, August 31, 1974. The preparation of this paper was supported by grant 73-NI-04-0002 from the National Institute of Law Enforcement Assistance Administration, United States Department of Justice. The fact that the National Institute of Law Enforcement and Criminal Justice furnished financial support to the activity described in this publication does not necessarily indicate the concurrence of the Institute in the statements or conclusions contained therein. The author wishes to thank Jonnie H. McLeod, M.D. for her contribution to this research effort.

REFERENCES

Lewis, Jerry M., Gossett, John T., and Phillips, Virginia Austin, "Evaluation of a drug prevention program," *Hospital and Community Psychiatry*, 23, No. 4 (April, 1972), 124-126.
National Commission on Marihuana and Drug Abuse, *Drug Use in America: Problem in Perspective*, Washington: U.S. Government Printing Office, March, 1973.
Swisher, John D. and Crawford, Jr., James L., "An evaluation of a short-term drug education program," *The School Counselor* (March, 1971), 265-272.
Weaver, Sue C. and Tennant, Jr., Forest S., "Effectiveness of drug education programs for secondary school students," *American Journal of Psychiatry*, 130, N. 7 (July 1973), 812-814.

CHAPTER 9

Cost-Benefit Analysis and Program Target Populations: The Narcotics Addiction Treatment Case

IRVING LEVESON

THE APPROACH

While cost-benefit analysis offers a potentially valuable tool for public decision-making on problems of human resources, as well as other program areas, its use in practice has been limited in significant part because of empirical difficulties which can be overcome. In a commonly used version, a set of alternatives is ranked according to the ratio of benefits to costs. Projects with the highest ratios are chosen first and the number of projects included is determined by a budget constraint. The framework is quite general. It says nothing about what should be defined as a project. If a program exhibits diminishing returns to scale, it is necessary only to treat successive increments as separate projects. If programs interact so that success depends on the combinations undertaken, increments of various combinations can be treated as separate projects. Definition of the array of alternatives is left to the analyst who is aware of the context in which the conclusions are to be used.

The situation in practice is quite different. The information demands of a full analysis are costly and difficult to meet and the number of alternatives that can be considered becomes limited. As a consequence, cost-benefit analysis has been

151

used rather infrequently as a formal tool, although it has gained in use as a way of thinking about problems. Empirical cost-benefit studies have too often considered only one specification of a program which is only one of a number of similar alternatives. Each program is assumed to have a fixed size and target population (or the question of target population is ignored entirely) and a single benefit/cost ratio is computed for the purpose of comparison with other programs. Relatively little attention has been given to the choices which must be made within program areas.

In comparing alternatives within a program area, it is necessary to take into consideration both variations in service and variations in the population being served. Ideally, we would like to know the ratio of benefits to costs for successive increments of resources to each combination of type of service and type of beneficiary. Combinations of service and beneficiary types will differ in benefit-cost ratio because of a number of factors. Population groups will differ in the extent of success. Here, the amount of improvement has to be measured relative to what would have happened in the absence of service, and this will often require separate calculations for different client groups. There will often be important differences in the value to be attached to a given amount of improvement. This can arise because of factors such as a positive value for efforts which redistribute well-being to less fortunate groups or differences in the period of time in which the gains can be expected to be maintained.

When complete information is lacking, a number of modifications of the methodology are possible. If we wish to compare two programs using different treatment methods serving different population groups, it would be possible to adjust the benefit-cost ratio of the first differences in ease of treatment and value of success which would be expected if it were to serve the second population group. This would make it possible to use information from the two programs to compare treatment variations within a given population. Similarly, if we would adjust the benefit-cost ratio of the first to the level expected were we to shift to the second method of treatment, it would then be possible to assess the effect of varying the population served within the second method of treatment.

If the way in which parameters of the cost-benefit model vary systematically with population characteristics is known, it is possible to go further and apply optimization models to the problem of determining the target population for each program which maximizes a set of criteria.

One further modification of the formal framework should be noted. Frequently in trying to make benefit-cost comparisons among programs, important information is missing. The approach used with limited information is a sensitivity analysis. Rather than rely on point estimates, we ask what the values of the missing information would have to be in order for the decision to change. A judgment is then made about whether the missing values are likely to be greater or less than the critical levels. This judgment normally requires much less knowledge than would be required for an exact value.

The application of these considerations is developed in the analysis of narcotics addiction treatment programs. Special attention is paid to the efficacy of serving persons of different ages. The next section considers the basic cost-benefit model, introducing the number of years of addiction remaining as a benefit criterion along with the probability of successful withdrawal. The section which follows examines the empirical evidence on age patterns of addiction and treatment and their implications for program evaluation. The application of the analysis is then illustrated for the problems of choosing among programs and for choice of population targets within programs.

THE UNDERLYING COST-BENEFIT MODEL

The benefit to society of having one less addict[1] depends on the number of years that the addict would have remained addicted without assistance. Because of a finite life expectancy and the possibility that many persons "mature out" of addiction as they grow older, the number of years of addiction remaining is greater for younger addicts. The number of remaining years of addiction is represented by 1.

The benefit of a reduction of a man-year of addiction (b_{ij}) are represented as a function of age (i) as well as the number of years (j) of addiction remaining.[2] Future benefits are discounted by an appropriate rate (r). The full expression for the benefits of $N = \Sigma_i N_i$ persons withdrawing from addiction is given by summing over individuals with different ages and numbers of years of addiction remaining:

$$B = \sum_{i=1}^{n} \sum_{j=1}^{l} \frac{N_{ij} l_j b_{ij}}{(1+r)^j} \tag{1}$$

Equation 1 can be greatly simplified. First, we assume that the number of years of addiction remaining is solely a function of age. Therefore we can write:

$$B = \sum_{j=1}^{l} \frac{N_j l_j b_j}{(1+r)^j} \tag{2}$$

Now we examine the assumptions implicitly required to use simpler measures of success than the full expression in Equation 2. Most studies ignore differences

---

[1] The term addict is used to imply users of hard drugs whether or not physiologically or psychologically addicted.

[2] One study of addicts with a mean age 30.7 showed a mean age of most arrests of 22.8. See Greenfield, 1967.

among age groups in annual benefits per addict successfully treated. The effectiveness measure becomes

$$E = \sum_{j=1}^{l} \frac{N_j l_j}{(1 + r)^j} \tag{3}$$

where $B = bE$. The most commonly used measure of success is the proportion (σ) of persons (A) admitted to treatment who successfully withdraw. The reduction in the number of addicts is $N = A\sigma$. If we compared different programs treating the same types of people, b_1 would equal b_2 and l_1 would equal l_2, so that σ, the probability of successful withdrawal, would be sufficient to gauge success. When age differs, use of this measure is equivalent to assuming that

$$\sum_{j=1}^{l} \frac{l_j}{(1 + r)^j} = 1 \tag{4}$$

as well as ignoring all differences in benefits per man-year of addiction averted. Sigma gauges success by the number of addicts successfully withdrawing without regard to length of time they would have been addicted. In doing so, it overemphasizes very immediate gains.

The measure of success which we would wish to maximize if the goal were to minimize the average number of addicts over a period of time is *the number of man-years of addiction averted,* or $M = Nl$. This can be derived from Equation 3 as:

$$M = \sum_{j=1}^{l} N_j l_j \tag{5}$$

where $r = 0$ and $B = bM$. This measure is particularly simple to use. However, it overemphasizes benefits which are deferred in time. If we wish to take into account that we value benefits today more than those which will not be received for many years, it is necessary to discount future benefits by an appropriate discount rate (r). The measure which does this is the discounted number of man-years of addiction averted, designated as E as defined in Equation 3.[3]

---

[3]If we make the assumption that the ratio of the benefits per man-year of addiction averted to the discount function is an inverse function of age

$$\frac{b_j}{(1 + r)^j} = \frac{k}{a} \quad \text{then}$$

$$B = \sum_{j=1}^{l} \frac{k}{a} l_j N_j$$

$$B = \frac{k}{a} M$$

The benefits of reducing addiction are proportional to the number of man-years of addiction averted and inversely related to the age of those assisted.

Next we consider cost-effectiveness. Where l is used, a discounted l could easily be substituted. Let individuals going through a program either be treated successfully at a cost c_s or unsuccessfully at a cost c_u. The average cost (c_t) of treating an addict in a program having a proportion successfully treated of σ is:

$$c_t = \sigma c_s + (1 - \sigma) c_u{}^4 \qquad (6)$$

The cost of treating A addicts is Ac_t, so that the cost per successfully treated addict is:

$$\frac{Ac_t}{\sigma A} = \frac{c_t}{\sigma}$$

Designating the cost per successfully treated addict as c, from Equation 6 we have:

$$c = c_s + \left(\frac{1 - \sigma}{\sigma}\right) c_u \qquad (7)$$

As the proportion successfully treated increases, cost per success falls because the costs of relatively fewer unsuccessful cases are included.

The ratio of the cost of addicts admitted to treatment to the number of man-years of addiction averted (cost-effectiveness ratio) is

$$\frac{c_t A}{M} \cong \frac{\sigma c_s + (1 - \sigma) c_u}{\sigma l} \qquad (8)$$

Assume that programs with a larger l have a lower σ. If across programs σ is proportional to l, the ratio of the cost-effectiveness ratios is the same as the ratio of the costs per person treated. If σ varies more than l, the costs per person treated would have to be lower in the programs with the higher l for them to compare favorably with the others. If c_u is small relative to c_s or σ is large

$$\frac{c_t A}{M} \simeq \frac{c_s}{l} \qquad (9)$$

Variations in the value attached to averting a man-year of addiction could similarly be taken into account.

---

[4] The model could easily be extended to allow for some positive benefit for nonsuccesses due to a period of withdrawal prior to recidivism.

NUMBER OF ADDICTS AGE 20-24   NUMBER OF ADDICTS BY AGE

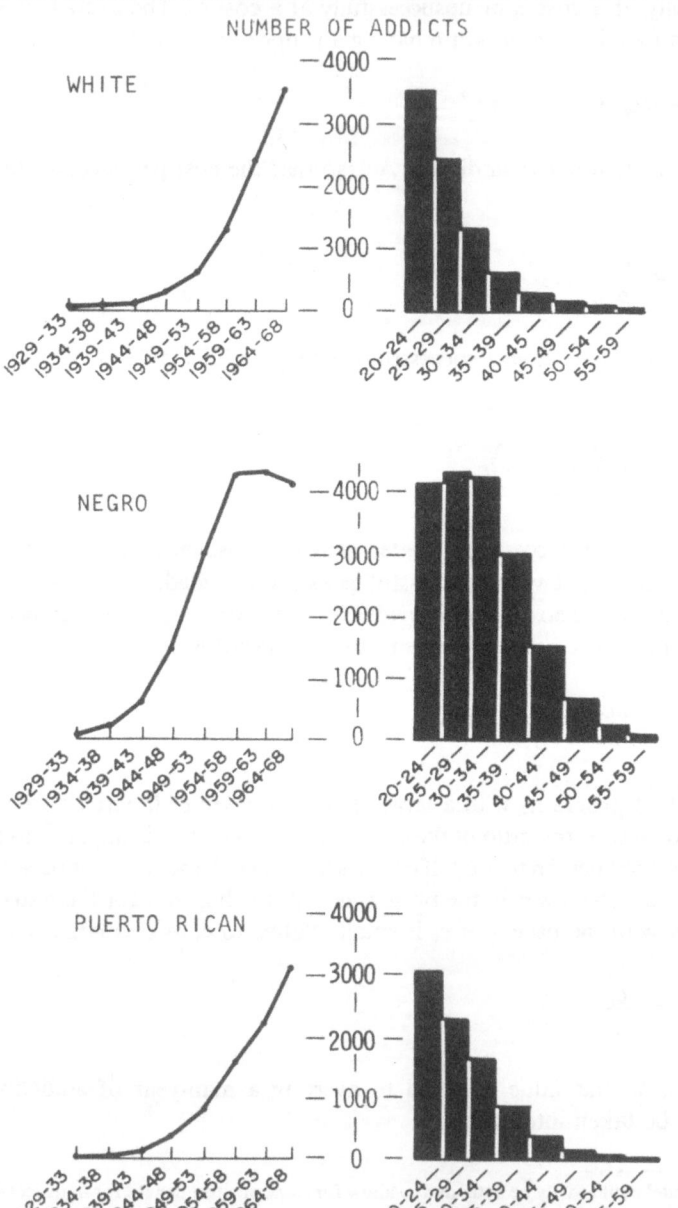

Fig. 1. Number of New Addicts Required to Produce the Current Age Distribution Assuming No Maturation.

EMPIRICAL EVIDENCE ON AGE DIFFERENCES

The Maturation Hypothesis

The age distribution of addicts shows a sharp decline after age 30-34 for Negroes and earlier for whites and Puerto Ricans, as indicated in data from the New York City Narcotics Register for 1967. The leading explanation is the "maturation hypothesis" of Charles Winnick, which states that addicts tend to "mature out" of addiction as they get older (Winnick, 1962). Interpretations of the maturation phenomenon are primarily psychological. A number of other explanations are possible. Employment opportunities may improve with age. Penalties for crimes committed to finance drug use rise with the number of offenses and the probability of apprehension and conviction may rise as a criminal becomes known. The high mortality of addicts may result in their disappearance. Moreover, the pattern may simply be the result of a rapid growth in the number of addicts with the newest addicts entering at the youngest ages.

For the age patterns to have been produced by growth in the number of addicts, they would have had to have been produced by rates of growth in the number of addicts over time which are highly implausible.[5] Available data, while scant, do not give too much credence to the mortality explanation. Whatever the explanation, it would seem that the maturation pattern is a real one, and hence age patterns can provide a valuable basis for measuring the length of the benefit period. The age distribution of heroin users listed on the Narcotics Register is shown for each ethnic group in the right panel of Figure 1. The data on age groups below age 20 are omitted since new addicts take some time to become known to authorities. If there were no maturation, the time path of the number of 20- to 24-year-old addicts would be the mirror image of the age distribution. This is shown in the left panels. It is clear that denial of the maturation hypothesis implies that very rapid growth in the number of addicts must have occurred in the past. While little information is available on the number of addicts over time and the accuracy of the data is poor, the implied growth rates are far higher than suggested by any data or than observers typically believe to be the case.

In Figure 2, we have computed the time paths of the number of 20- to 24-year-old addicts, alternatively assuming 3 percent and 6 percent annual rates of maturation. The implied long-run growth rates of the number of addicts are still far too high to appear reasonable. The age profile of Blacks peaks about 10 years after whites. Some observers have noted an unusual increase in the number of addicts after the Korean War. The patterns of changes over time suggest this is

---

[5]Authors of longitudinal studies of selected groups of addicts have claimed evidence that there is little if any maturation. However, these studies have tended to consider addicts relatively few of whom were at ages at which maturation is likely to occur. For example, see Ball and Snarr (1969).

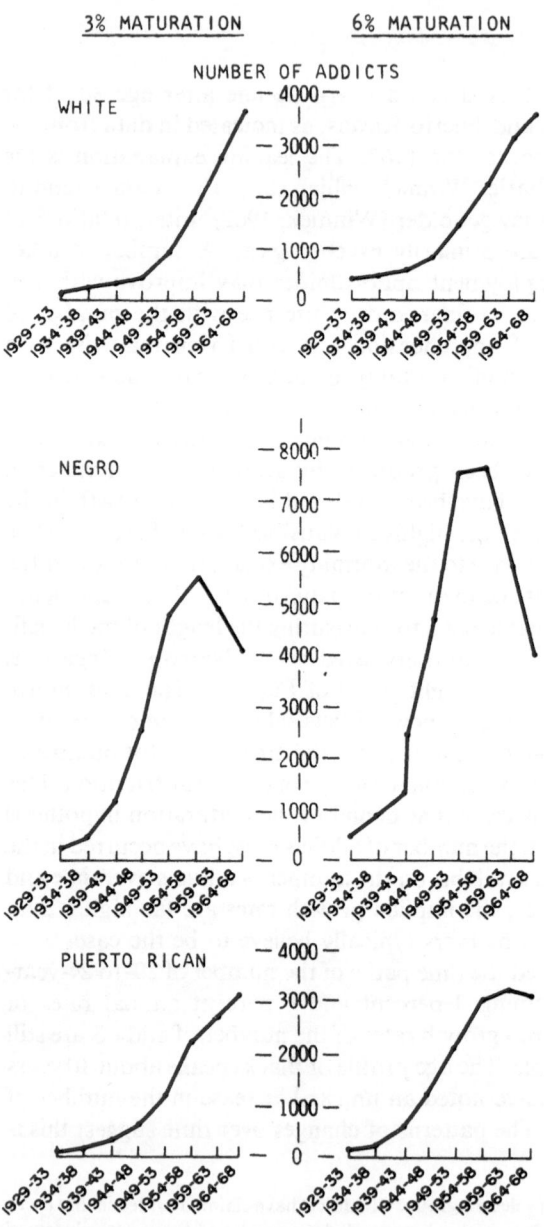

Fig. 2. Number of Addicts Age 20-24 Required to Produce the Current Age Distribution Assuming 3% and 6% Maturation.

possible, but it may have applied to Blacks and not whites. The timing of the derived increase in new Black addicts is suspiciously coincident with the timing of the large rise in unemployment rates of Blacks relative to whites around 1956 exhibited by national data. An alternative explanation is that Blacks become addicts at older ages. Barring these explanations, the data would imply that Blacks begin to mature when they are relatively older.

Table 1. Average Annual Rates of Maturation of Heroin Abusers Between Successive Five-Year Age Intervals Consistent With Alternative Assumptions About The Rate of Growth of the Number of Abusers Over Time, By Ethnic Group, New York City

Change Between Age Intervals	Whites	Negroes	Puerto Ricans
Assuming No Growth*			
20-24 and 25-29	9%	†%	5%
25-29 and 30-34	12	1	7
30-34 and 35-39	14	6	14
35-39 and 40-44	19	14	16
40-44 and 45-49	15	18	21
45-49 and 50-54	11	21	24
50-54 and 55-59	7	19	9
Assuming 3 Percent Growth*			
20-24 and 25-29	6	†	3
25-29 and 30-34	9	†	4
30-34 and 35-39	11	3	11
35-39 and 40-44	16	12	14
40-44 and 45-49	12	16	19
45-49 and 50-54	8	19	22
50-54 and 55-59	4	16	6
Assuming 6 Percent Growth*			
20-24 and 25-29	3	†	†
25-29 and 30-34	3	†	1
30-34 and 35-39	9	1	8
35-39 and 40-44	14	9	11
40-44 and 45-49	10	13	16
45-49 and 50-54	6	16	20
50-54 and 55-59	2	14	3

*Based on assumption about the growth rate in the number of 20 to 24-year-old heroin abusers over time.

†The number of heroin abusers either increases or declines less rapidly than the assumed rate of growth, implying a negative maturation rate.

Source: Based on data in Zili Amsel et al., "The Narcotics Register: Development of a Case Register," paper presented at the 31st Annual Meeting of the Committee on Problems of Drug Dependence, National Academy of Sciences—National Research Council, Palo Alto, California, February 25, 1969, Table V.

An alternative way of looking at the data is to determine what annual maturation rate between age intervals are implied by alternative assumptions about the rate of growth of the number of addicts over time. Calculations based on assumptions of no growth, 3 percent growth and 6 percent growth are shown in Table 1. With any assumption these rates are quite large. The number of Puerto Rican addicts may have been growing more rapidly than the others because of more rapid population growth in the age groups with high addiction. It is interesting to note that the pattern of maturation rates for Puerto Ricans based on the assumption of 6 percent growth is nearly identical with the Negro pattern assuming no growth. However, both of these patterns may differ from whites because of changes over time. Therefore, we cannot refute the simple assumption that maturation rates are the same for all ethnic groups, and equal to the white rates.

Years of Addiction Remaining

In order to determine the gains from successfully treating younger addicts relative to those of treating older addicts, we have made use of the New York City Narcotics Register data to derive the average number of years of addiction remaining between the ages 22 and 42. These figures reflect life expectancy as well as maturation. The data are shown for each ethnic group based on alternative assumptions about the growth of the number of addicts over time in Figure 3. The calculations were limited to age 42 because of difficulties imposed by the open-ended age interval. The larger average number of years of addiction remaining for younger persons is apparent. The average number of years of addiction remaining appears to be higher for Blacks and Puerto Ricans than for whites at the youngest ages, with the reverse the case among older addicts.

If effectiveness is measured by the number of man-years of addiction averted, a program treating 33-year-old whites would have to have a probability of successful withdrawal 1 1/3 times the probability of one treating 23-year-old whites, in order to be equally effective, based on the no growth assumption.

Age Differences in Ease of Treatment

The simplest available way of determining whether some groups are more successfully treated by one method or another is to examine evidence on the success of a given program on different groups. Such data has recently become available for the New York City Methadone Program. The relevant information is reproduced as Figure 4. The curves show the characteristic decline in the proportion continuing in the program with length of time since entry. The

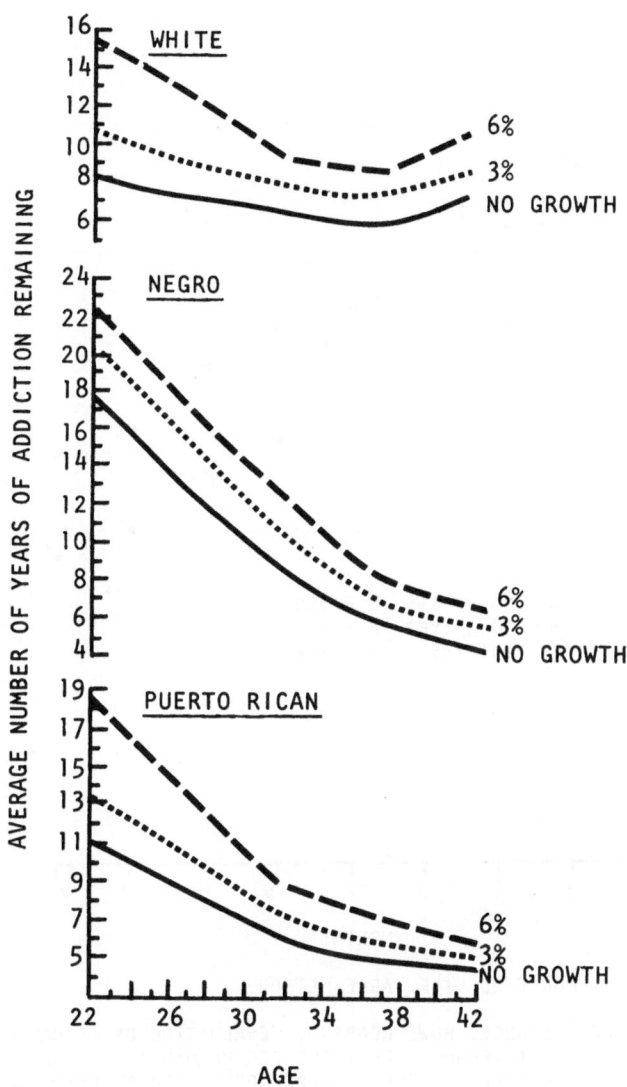

Fig. 3. Average Number of Years of Addiction Remaining by Age and Ethnic Groups Assuming Alternative Rates of Growth.

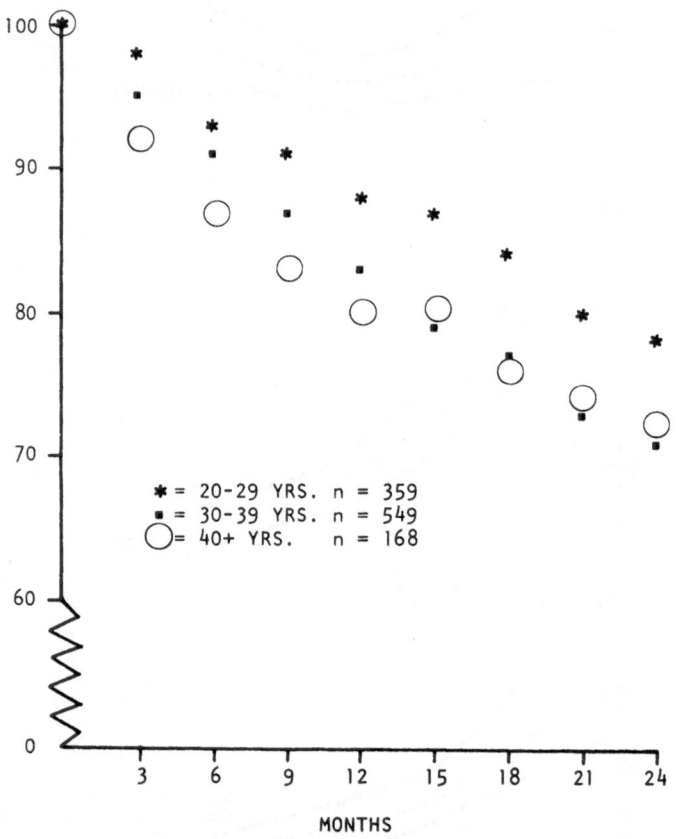

NOTE: MODIFIED LIFE TABLE METHOD.

SOURCE: FRANCES ROWE GEARING, "EVALUATION OF METHADONE
MAINTENANCE TREATMENT FOR HEROIN ADDICTION: A
PROGRESS REPORT." PAPER PRESENTED AT EPIDEMIOLOGY
SECTION OF THE AMERICAN PUBLIC HEALTH ASSOCIATION,
NOVEMBER 1969, FIGURE 6.

Fig. 4. Methadone Maintenance Treatment Program Probability of Remaining in Program by Month for Men by Age of Time of Admission as of September 15, 1969.

principal reasons for discharge include drug abuse, alcohol use, arrest, and voluntary withdrawal. Contrary to expectations, there is tendency for continuation to be greatest among the youngest addicts.

However, these results cannot be used in raw form. Rates of continuation may seem higher where rates of maturing out are high. Table 1 indicated differences in maturation rates between 20- to 29-year-olds and 30- to 39-year-olds of 5-10 percent per year. Figure 4 indicates that the younger group remained in the program by about 7 percentage points more after two years.

Whites age 40 or more have lower maturation than whites age 30-39, with the reverse true for Blacks and Puerto Ricans. If maturation were the cause of differences in continuation rates, when ethnic groups were aggregated, we would expect to find no clear difference in continuation rates between the age groups, and in fact there is none. Another factor hinting at the effect of maturation on measured continuation rates is that Blacks entering the Methadone Program are four years older than whites, a difference which cannot be unlike the ethnic difference in average age at maturation.

It appears that after differences in "apparent success" due to differences in rates of maturation are taken into account, younger persons seem to have about the same tendency to discontinue participation in the program as persons of other ages.

The evidence on differences among age groups in the benefits of successful treatment and the chances for successful treatment (a) indicates that differences in the prevalence of opiate use among age groups reflects some sort of maturation (and/or mortality) since without maturation they imply implausible patterns in the number of users over time, (b) provides implications for the average number of years of addiction remaining by ethnic group based on age patterns under alternative assumptions about past rates of growth of addiction, and (c) suggests that the young may do about the same as older persons in the program if maturation accounts for part of the observed differences in continuation.

A CURSORY LOOK AT MAJOR PROGRAMS

Virtually any program will pay in terms of benefits to the non-addict population. Even if we incarcerate persons at a cost of over $8,000 per year for several years, if crime of $10,000 to $20,000 per person per year is averted (see the program can be justified (see Leveson [Chapter 5] and Holahan [1970]). However, this calculation does not consider that, even with a high payoff, funds for addiction services may be limited, and it does not take into account any factor for undesirability of involuntary incarceration. While it may be clear that the payoff to addiction programs in general is very high, there is still a major issue as to what proportion of the addict population can be dealt with by each approach.

As of the end of 1969, there were about 11,000 New York City addicts in treatment programs. In addition, there were about 5,000 in pre-trial detention and others serving prison terms or on parole. Nearly all treatment funding came from the New York State Narcotic Addiction Control Commission which had an operating budget of $38 million per year and a $200 million capital construction program. By 1972, the number in treatment had risen to 50,000, and the budget of the New York City Addiction Services Agency exceeded $100 million. The three largest programs for the treatment of drug addicts in New York City are the program of the New York State Narcotics Addiction Control Commission, the Methadone Maintenance Program, and the Phoenix House therapeutic community program of New York City's Addiction Services Agency.

The State program combines voluntary or involuntary incarceration with therapeutic and rehabilitation services for up to five years, followed by an aftercare phase involving surveillance. The program, depending strongly on court and parental coercion, has suffered abscondance rates of over one-third per year and high rates of recidivism. However, it has had some success in moving persons from an institutional setting into aftercare. Furthermore, it is the only one of the three largest programs to have given primary attention to younger addicts. One-third of the persons in the program are under age 20 and two-thirds are under age 25. The availability of rehabilitation services under the program has been limited. At the end of 1971, there were 16,000 addicts in the program.

The Methadone Program uses the drug Methadone, itself addicting but providing no "high," to block the effect of opiates. After a few weeks of withdrawal, the drug is administered orally on an outpatient basis of an indefinite period of time. There were about 2,000 addicts under treatment in 1969, the period for which much of our data apply. Subsequent efforts led to an increase in the number of persons in Methadone programs in New York City to 17,000 in 1972. This program tends to concentrate on older addicts as indicated by comparisons with the Narcotics Register for September, 1969:

	Methadone Program	Narcotics Register
Less than 25	10%	33%
25–34	51	41
35 and over	39	16

The Methadone Program has provided regular public evaluation reports. The evidence of high retention rates, improvement in employment experience, and reduced criminality have led to a belief that this is the most effective method currently available.

The Methadone Program reported about a 70 percent success rate for persons on drug maintenance for 36 months. Lack of success in that program reflects both voluntary and involuntary termination stemming from factors such as criminal behavior and alcoholism.

The state program reported that after its first 21 months of operations, 44 percent of the 1,893 persons returned to the community had not resumed drug use. Thirty percent were returned to the rehabilitation center after it was discovered that they were re-using narcotics, and 26 percent could not longer be located (warrants were issued against them).[6] In view of the fact that the program had only 188 persons on aftercare after its first year and 836 after 21 months, the average length of time in the community would have to have been substantially less than one year. In view of the short time, the program's experience is discouraging.

A study of a roughly similar program, that of the California Rehabilitation Center at Corona, found that 35 percent were in good standing (or had been removed from the program while in good standing) one year after release. After three years, the figure had fallen to 19 percent (Kramer and Bass, [1968]). There is nothing in the experience of the New York State program to date to indicate it is doing any better than this.

We are now in a position to compare programs on the *assumption that they continue to treat the same types of people as they now treat with the same degree of success.* If we compare the benefits of the Methadone program designated by subscript 1 relative to the state program designated by subscript 2, we have:

$$\frac{B_1}{B_2} = \frac{b_1 \sigma_1 l_1}{b_2 \sigma_2 l_2} \tag{10}$$

The number of persons admitted to each program is assumed to be the same. Assuming the California experience to be applicable to New York State, σ_1/σ_2 equals about .7/.2 or $3\frac{1}{2}$.

The mean ages and corresponding years of addiction remaining for the three major programs are as follows:

	Age	Approximate Years Remaining
Narcotic Addiction Commission	25	13
Addiction Services Agency	27	11
Methadone Maintenance	32	8

---

[6]New York State (1969). The Commission did not release comparable figures in its second annual report. In the week of January 25-31, 1970, only 48 percent were known to be gainfully occupied.

The age distribution of the Methadone program implies that a successful withdrawal is worth only two-thirds as much in the Methadone program as in the state program because of the difference in man-years of addiction averted. If the years of addiction remaining were discounted, this difference would be modified somewhat.

The value to society of treating the kinds of persons treated by the state program may be higher than those treated with Methadone. There is some evidence that older addicts commit fewer crimes. However, younger addicts can be expected to remain on drugs longer, with greater adverse effects on health. Furthermore, treatment of younger addicts may have greater benefits of preventing other persons from being induced to use drugs. Nevertheless, it does not appear likely that these factors are so large as to outweigh the huge difference in the proportion of addicts who successfully withdraw. When allowance is made for the greater disadvantage of the involuntary nature of the state program than the dependence on Methadone, the relative advantage of the Methadone program becomes even greater.

In the past, the state program required over $8,000 in operating costs alone per man-year of incarceration, and currently employs nearly one person for every addict in residential or aftercare activities. Completion of the program probably requires an average of about $15,000 per person. For a comparable cost, the Methadone program could provide detoxification and drug maintenance for more than a decade. After that time, it may be possible for maturation effects to be substituted for drug maintenance.

What costs and benefits are both considered the evidence clearly indicates that Methadone is preferred to the New York State program.

CHOICE OF AGE GROUP WITHIN A PROGRAM

Selecting age groups for treatment so as to maximize the number of man-years of addiction averted is equivalent to minimizing the number of addicts. If the success of treatment were the same at each age, we would concentrate on the youngest addicts who have the greatest number of years of addiction remaining. On the other hand, if the number of years of addiction remaining were the same at each age and success of treatment were greater for older persons, we would concentrate on the oldest addicts. (We are defining success net of any normal maturation tendencies.) Here we consider the optimal age when variations in both years of addiction remaining and success of treatment are taken into account.

The number of man-years of addiction averted for a program is given by

$$M = A\sigma l \tag{11}$$

For simplicity, we assume that the average number of years of addiction remaining in a program can be represented as a proportion (p) of the difference between some fixed age (a*) and the average age (a) of persons being treated.

$$1 = p(a^* - a) \tag{12}$$

Thus if a* is age 40 and p = .6, addicts age 20 would be expected to remain addicted for another 12 years on the average while those who were still addicted at age 30 would be expected to remain addicted for another 6 years. We further assume that the rate of success in withdrawal from addiction can be represented by a linear function of age

$$\sigma = s + ta, \tag{13}$$

where t > 0.
Combining these equations we have

$$M = Asp(a^* - a) + Atap(a^* + a) \tag{14}$$

Multiplying through and differentiating with respect to age

$$dM/da = Ata^*p - Asp - 2Atpa \tag{15}$$

The second derivative is

$$d^2M/da^2 = -2Atp \tag{16}$$

which, since A, t and p are positive, is negative indicating a maximum. Setting the first derivative equal to zero and solving, we derive the optimal level of a

$$a = \frac{a^*}{2} - \frac{s}{2t} \tag{17}$$

One inference that can be drawn from this result is that the effect of age differences in the success rate on the optimal age is important. If, for example, s were −.3 and t were .03, indicating a success rate of .4 at age 20, and .7 at age 30, the s/2t term would add five years to the optimal age. If s is positive, however, the optimal age is reduced. For example, if s = .2 and t = .02, indicating success of .6 at age 20 and .8 at age 30, the optimal age would be reduced by five years.

With the functional form we have chosen for l, p does not enter into the result since it does not change the terms of trade between age groups. Unfortunately, we have little information with which to determine a*. Our curves of years of addiction remaining suggest that over the range of ages 22-32 the curves could be approximated by an a* at about 40, with different p's for each ethnic group. In that age range, a figure of age 20 for a*/2 would be valid. This is very approximate of course.

If a*/2 were as high as 25 and a function such as $\sigma = -.3 + .03a$ were approximately correct, we would come out with an optimal age very close to the average age now being treated in the Methadone program. If, instead, as the program claims, success varies little with age so that a function such as $\sigma = .2 + .02t$ is appropriate, then to corroborate the ages now treated we would need an a* of around 70 which is completely impossible. Even if a* is as high as 50, $s \simeq .2$ and $t \simeq .02$, then the Methadone program should be concentrating on persons as much as 10 years younger than they are now, even though the proportion successfully withdrawing would be lower if it did. This would take into account the likelihood that addiction will be prevented for a larger number of years when the young withdraw, rather than relying on the more visible success rate (σ) alone.

The possible reduction in the number of addicts by shifting services to younger age groups can be easily seen in the case where σ does not vary by age at all. The savings are then equal to the difference in l. On the basis of Figure 3, it appears that present programs could increase their impact on the number of addicts by 50 percent or more by concentrating on the young.

DISCUSSION

The results of this analysis are illustrative and suggestive rather than definitive. They tend to support the efficacy of the Methadone program relative to the state program, if the goal is to minimize the number of addicts. However, they raise serious questions about the merits of the Methadone program's practice of treating a disproportionate number of older addicts.

The specific methodologies employed to deal with age may be particularly appropriate for areas such as mental health, physical rehabilitation and crime where processes of maturation and deterioration occur. Age is a special characteristic in its relationship to time, but there are many characteristics with which success and value can vary.

The general approach in which characteristics of population served are taken into account in considering costs, effectiveness and value of success has been demonstrated. The ability to obtain a true picture when we compare programs or to achieve the maximum amount of impact from a given program can be greatly influenced by taking into account population as well as treatment factors.

ACKNOWLEDGMENTS

This study was initiated while at the RAND Corporation. The comments of Zili Amsel, Sidney Leveson and Clarence Teng are appreciated.

Most of the paper was originally published in *The American Journal of Economics and Sociology,* April 1973. The permission of the editors to reprint the material is appreciated.

REFERENCES

Ball, John C. and Snarr, Richard, "A test of the maturation hypothesis with respect to opiate addiction," paper presented at the Thirty-First Annual Meeting of the Committee on Problems of Drug Dependence, National Academy of Services—National Research Council, Palo Alto, Calif., February 25 and 26, 1969.

Greenfield, Bernard, "The Riverside Study—Ten Years Late," paper prepared for the New York City Department of Health, Health Research Training Program, Summer, 1967.

Holohan, John, *The Economics of Drug Addiction in Washington, D.C.: A Model for Estimation of Costs and Benefits of Treatment and Rehabilitation,* Report No. 33, District of Columbia Department of Corrections, October, 1970.

Kramer, John and Bass, Richard A., "Civil Commitment for Addicts: The California Program," Report of the Committee on Problems of Drug Dependency of the National Academy of Sciences and the National Research Council, 1968.

New York State, "Report of the Narcotic Addiction Control Commission for the First Twenty-One-Month Period," 1969.

Winnick, Charles, "Maturing out of narcotic addiction," *Bulletin of Narcotics,* U.N. Department of Social Affairs, 14, No. 1 (1962).

CHAPTER 10

Employing the Ex-Addict: An Experiment in Supported Work

LUCY N. FRIEDMAN

Wildcat Service Corporation was established in 1972. Its aim was to explore the possibility that ex-addicts—traditionally viewed as unemployable and a threat to society—could become a resource to society by developing work habits in a supported setting.

Wildcat was the most ambitious of a series of supported work projects started by the Vera Institute of Justice. Vera, a nonprofit organization located in New York City and concerned with criminal justice reform, has been trying for the past fifteen years to break the tie of addiction, crime, and unemployment. After considering various approaches, the Vera staff came to believe that placement in the low stress jobs might work as a strategy for rehabilitating addicts. Specifically, Vera sought to answer four questions:

- Could a work environment be designed in which chronically unemployed persons with drug histories would work productively?
- Would work experience in such an environment prepare employees for the competitive world?
- Would employment (either in the special environment or the competitive market) lift the participant out of the cycle of welfare, addiction, and crime?
- Could such a low-stress working environment be created so that investment in the program was returned to the taxpayer?

Seeking answers, Vera staff studied European sheltered workshops for the handicapped and drew upon experience from its own programs with accused persons, alcoholics, and ex-addicts[1] to develop the concept of "supported work." Supported work derives from the premise that persons not previously successful in the job market can learn skills, develop good work habits, and build self-confidence while earning a wage—if they are placed in job settings where management and peers are sensitive to their special problems. To test the feasibility of this idea, Vera conducted a series of pilot projects[2] and then created the Wildcat Service Corporation in 1972. Since then nearly 4,000 ex-addicts and ex-offenders referred from drug treatment programs and correctional facilities have worked at Wildcat. The Corporation now employs 1,200 ex-addicts and ex-offenders, 90 percent of whom provide services to the City of New York: 35 percent work in maintenance, 14 percent in construction, 45 percent as clerks or social service paraprofessionals, and 6 percent as messengers.

Wildcat, unlike many of the European agencies examined, is a transitional rather than a permanent employer. By providing chronically unemployed ex-addicts and ex-offenders some employment stability in a supportive environment, it aims to prepare them for the regular job market.

In an attempt to answer the questions that Wildcat was created to address, Vera established a research team to study supported work and its impact on the participants. The research team has three strategies: an examination of the day-to-day operations of Wildcat; a four-year controlled study comparing approximately 300 qualified applicants offered jobs at Wildcat with 300 qualified applicants who were not; and cost-benefit analyses.

THE PEOPLE WILDCAT EMPLOYS

Eligibility criteria for Wildcat were designed to provide supported employment for ex-addicts who had a history of failure in the marketplace but who had demonstrated a desire to change their lives. Accordingly, ex-addict applicants may not have worked at one job for more than six months in the last two years but have had to be in drug treatment for at least three months. Other criteria include being 18 years of age, a New York City resident, and receiving public assistance.

About three-quarters of Wildcat workers have not worked a day during the six months before they enter Wildcat. Over 90 percent do not have bank accounts.

---

[1]The Manhattan Court Employment project, Project Renewal (a subsidiary of the Manhattan Bowery Project), and the Addiction Research and Treatment Corporation.

[2]Vera established the Pioneer Messenger Service which employed ex-addicts, ex-offenders, and ex-alcoholics and also staffed City Off-Track Betting offices with ex-addicts.

Over 50 percent lack previous job training. Literacy levels are low; Wildcatters have been schooled an average of 10 years but average only fifth grade scores on arithmetic exams. Ninety percent are black or Hispanic men.

Wildcatters are handicapped in obtaining jobs by their criminal and addiction histories. The average worker is 31 years old with a record of eight arrests and four convictions. The mean age of first addiction to drugs is 19. Seventy-two percent are referred to Wildcat from methadone programs and 18 percent from drug-free programs. These referrals—who constitute 90 percent of employees—have spent an average of 13 months in drug programs before coming to Wildcat. The remaining 10 percent are referred from correctional facilities or are awaiting trial; about two-thirds of these persons have addiction histories.

Unpromising as these statistics are for finding jobs in the competitive labor market, even they do not adequately convey the tangle of problems that many Wildcat employees carry with them when they arrive at Wildcat. Addiction and criminal history reflect more than unaccounted years on a job resume; they reflect an individual's history of destructiveness toward himself and society and a sense of anomie. As one Wildcat worker put it: "When I applied to Wildcat, I hadn't worked since '49 or '51 and I was definitely ingrained in nothing. I was coming off somewhat an alcoholic and tired. And when you're tired, you don't know what you're tired of 'cause you're resting all the time."

THE CHARACTER OF SUPPORTED WORK

Because of the employees' poor preparation for work, instability is tolerated at Wildcat within wider boundaries than in the nonsubsidized world. Dismissal is nearly always preceded by warnings, suspensions, and other intermediate measures. Workers are given occasional time off for court appearances or visits with parole officers and drug-treatment counselors. Wildcat also offers special supports to its workers such as vocational counseling and referrals to outside agencies for assistance with housing, legal, and health problems.

A number of structural devices were built into Wildcat to reduce stress and encourage steady work habits. For instance, workers are put in small crews to allow strong peer support. The crews are headed by foremen who have been promoted up from the entry-level ranks of ex-addicts, a policy that provides both a visible career path and first level supervisors who share the problems of crew members. Bonuses, raises, and promotions come more frequently than in normal job situations. Participants begin at a $95-a-week salary but become eligible for their first raises after eight weeks. (Top salary for crewmen is $115 a week; for foremen, $125 a week.) Standards for raises are gradually made more stringent to accustom the employee to the discipline demanded in nonsubsidized work.

Though support services, such as counseling or training are offered, the emphasis at Wildcat is on work. Work is seen as therapy and Wildcat is structured to resemble the nonsubsidized job world rather than a therapeutic community. Standards are set and employees are dismissed if they do not meet the standards. The Wildcat employee who was "ingrained in nothing" said it this way: "Wildcat took me out of (the 'tired syndrome') and I made my first move. Getting up in the morning was a problem for me, but it gave me a push. That's what Wildcat gave me; it gave me that kick in the butt I needed."

THE WORK WILDCAT DOES

Wildcat's work consists mainly of providing public services for New York City. For example, Wildcatters clean building facades and interior masonry, restore clipper ships, paint commercial and public establishments, paint no-parking zones at fire hydrants, exterminate vermin, maintain buildings and grounds at various agencies (including courthouses, district attorneys' offices, and police precinct houses), prepare architectural plans for microfilming, renovate firehouses, interpret for Spanish-speaking hospital patients, and plant trees in Brooklyn. In spring 1975 when a fire destroyed a large New York Telephone plant, Wildcat workers provided emergency messenger service to affected businesses.

There are constraints on the selection of job sites, among them the special needs of Wildcat workers. Wildcat tries to avoid taking extremely demeaning jobs that might reinforce the employees' sense of being locked into the lowest rungs of the economic ladder. Night work, too, is avoided because it impedes employees' efforts to reestablish family and community ties.

Attractive jobs are difficult to find, however. Some Civil Service agencies resist hiring Wildcatters because many see them as a threat to their own employees; they fear that the increasingly impoverished city government will replace regular workers with cheap Wildcat labor. Other jobs are blocked by trade and craft labor unions; still others by stereotypes and prejudiced attitudes. One prospective employer, a police officer, admitted, "I used to arrest kids just the way (the Wildcatters) looked. How could I have one of them working in my office?" The supervisor in one agency reported that women employees refused to use the bathrooms because they were afraid they would contract venereal disease from the Wildcat women they thought were prostitutes. Many agencies are reluctant to hire persons with criminal records, which excludes almost all Wildcatters. And finally, the search for attractive jobs is difficult because the typical Wildcatter lacks marketable skills.

Because of these constraints, the Wildcat staff sometimes have had to create new types of work for the crews, such as home delivery of food to the elderly, a serivce no other organization supplied.

Wildcat favors jobs that offer an opportunity for employees to "roll over" to permanent positions on the sponsoring agency's staff. And group, or crew, work is favored over individual placement; small crews not only afford peer support but are more easily supervised. Individual placements are made when work is particularly challenging, where agency supervision is strong, or where the opportunity for roll over is good. These individual placements are generally given to experienced Wildcatters.

THE FUNDING OF WILDCAT

Wildcat funding comes from diverse sources, reflecting the organization's multiple aims. For the 1975–76 fiscal year, the per-person cost has been $9,500, of which about $6,600 is paid to the employee in salary and fringe benefits.

The employees' salaries are put together from three types of income. Through an arrangement with the Social Security Administration, the welfare benefits (Supplemental Security Income) that employees would receive had they still been unemployed are directed into a Wildcat salary pool. These diverted welfare funds make up $2,400 of each Wildcatter's salary. Another $2,000 comes from contracts with local municipal and private agencies (about 70 percent of Wildcat's crew members provide reimbursable services to these agencies). The rest comes from contracts and grants from New York City's Department of Employment and the U.S. Department of Labor (both interested in developing employment skills), from the National Institute on Drug Abuse (primarily concerned with learning whether the cycle of drug abuse can be broken by providing ex-addicts with employment opportunities), and from the Law Enforcement Assistance Administration (concerned with crime control).

RESEARCH STUDIES OF WILDCAT

The Vera Institute research studies on how the program operated and its impact on participants began at the same time Wildcat did.[3] To assess any changes experienced by Wildcat employees, the researchers designed a controlled study. By lottery, half of the first 600 eligible applicants were offered a job at Wildcat (to form the experimental group) and half were not (to form the control group). Together these two groups are called the "Manhattan sample."

Since the beginning of the experiment in 1972, experimentals and controls have been interviewed every three months about their employment, welfare

---

[3]Research on Wildcat was funded by the Addiction Services Agency of New York City, the National Institute on Drug Abuse, and the Department of Employment of New York City.

dependence, living arrangements, criminal and drug experiences, and leisure-time activities. (To induce people not working at Wildcat to come in for interviews, $5 is paid for the quarterly session and $10 for the longer annual interview.) Self-reported data from the interviews have been verified through arrest records from the New York City Police Department. Data are available for about 85 percent of the experimental and control group participants through the second year.

Members of the experimental group include those still at Wildcat, those who never showed up for Wildcat, and those who have terminated from Wildcat—that is, were fired, resigned, or moved on to nonsubsidized jobs. One difficulty with the study design is that 11 percent of the accepted applicants never showed up for work. These "no-shows" remain in the experimental group but have never been exposed to the supported work program. And another 9 percent worked fewer than three months at Wildcat. Consequently, differences between controls and experimentals are diluted.

DO EX-ADDICTS MAKE GOOD WORKERS?

Wildcat's experience shows that ex-addicts and ex-offenders can work in a supportive environment. Absenteeism levels (approximately 9 percent) are higher than the national averages, but not so high as to interfere significantly with productivity.

In its first four years, 4,000 persons worked at Wildcat, staying an average of 12 months. On the average, one year after date of hire, 58 percent of the employees are no longer at Wildcat. By the end of a second year, three out of four are off the Wildcat payroll, and by the end of the third year, seven out of eight have left Wildcat. Of those 4,000, 1,200 are now employed at Wildcat, 541 have graduated to nonsubsidized jobs, 66 have returned to school, 1,079 were terminated with cause, 448 left for non-job-related reasons, and 666 resigned. Almost half of the employees who resign or are fired obtain other jobs.

Results from the controlled study in which the working pattern of experimentals was examined indicate that Wildcat significantly increased the proportion of ex-addicts who could be productively employed. One year after entry into the study, 70 percent of experimentals were working compared to 34 percent of controls. Although the difference had narrowed by the second year (62 percent of experimentals working compared to 41 percent of controls), it was still significant. In addition, more experimentals than controls worked at some time; they worked for longer time; and they earned more money (Table 1).

A series of productivity studies in which the Wildcat workers were observed and their output measured suggests that although productivity is not uniformly high, Wildcatters produce valuable and needed services. Productivity for

Table 1. First and Second-Year Employment and Income:
Manhattan Sample
(Self-Reported)

Employment and Income Data	Experimentals N = 199	Controls N = 217
Percentage Working at Some Time During Year		
First Year	92	51
Second Year	76	47
Mean Number of Weeks Worked		
First Year	39	12
Second Year	32	17
Mean Weekly Earnings of Those Who Worked		
First Year	$110	$ 98
Second Year	$125	$110

maintenance work is estimated at 80 percent of commercial standards; for clerical work, 78 percent; for painting, 20 percent.

FEEDING WORKERS BACK INTO THE NONSUBSIDIZED JOB MARKET

The number of persons graduating to nonsubsidized jobs has not been as high as originally anticipated, but graduates have been successfully employed after their Wildcat experience. Eighty-nine percent of randomly sampled Wildcat employees who moved on to nonsupported jobs (and for whom data are available) were still working after three months. Eighty percent retained their nonsupported jobs for at least a year.

Results from the controlled experiment show that those who participated in Wildcat's supported work program are more likely to be successful in the open market after leaving Wildcat than the controls who did not have an opportunity to work at Wildcat. Experimentals who graduated from Wildcat as well as those terminated work more weeks at higher average pay, and are fired less often from nonsubsidized jobs than are controls (Table 2).[4]

---

[4]These figures are based on participants' own reports. Attempts to verify self-reported employment data have revealed that self-reported job information from experimentals is more likely to be accurate than that from controls. This suggests that the differences in employment between controls and experimentals are greater than indicated here.

Table 2. Comparison of Experimentals and Controls
in NonSubsidized Employment

	Experimentals	Controls
Average number of weeks worked during two years after entering study	29 at non-subsidized jobs and 36 at Wildcat (N = 199)	29 (N = 217)
Mean Weekly Salary of those who worked*	$132 (N = 79)*	$106 (N = 115)†
Percent Fired*	44 (N = 79)*	59 (N = 115)†

*Post Wildcat experimentals.
†Controls who worked.

Until spring 1976 no time limit was imposed on employment at Wildcat. Wildcat management thought that Wildcatters would move on when they felt ready for nonsubsidized work. But experience has shown that employees are reluctant to leave supported work, partly because their employment prospects are uncertain and their confidence has not been bolstered by the shrinking job market. (Unemployment in New York City went from 6.5 percent in 1972 to 11.9 percent in 1975.) Too, many feel—appropriately, as it has turned out— unprepared for outside jobs. When Wildcat first began, it was thought that formal training was less important than instilling good work habits. Whatever training deemed necessary was to be done on the job. But the job development specialists at Wildcat discovered that many of the employees did not have sufficient skills for industry standards even though they had been doing well in supported work. This led to the creation of in-house training programs and more vocational counselors. The newly-imposed time limit on employment is increasing the demand for skills training and increasing pressure on employees to improve their skills. One Wildcatter who enrolled in an IBM-sponsored clerical training course said: "I'm not a young man and this is the last chance for me in the event that I ever make anything of myself, and hopefully by getting into Wildcat and IBM I was trying to get sort of a background so somebody might accept me, because before I had none."

DOES WILDCAT REHABILITATE?

The Vera Institute originally developed the program of supported work not simply to provide employment but to loosen the tie between addiction, unemployment and crime. And data from the controlled experiment, which compared ex-addicts who worked at Wildcat with similar persons who did not, indicate that the supported work program has made a positive but not consistent impact in the areas of dependence on public assistance, drug and alcohol use, criminal activity, and other living patterns.

Dependence on Public Assistance

Experimentals who have left Wildcat are less likely to receive public assistance than are controls (Table 3).

Experimentals who had left Wildcat and controls received approximately the same monthly stipends, however, a significantly smaller proportion of experimentals than controls were dependent on direct assistance two years after entering the study.

Drug Use

It was anticipated that drug use would decrease for experimentals as a consequence of more stable employment, the supportive work environment, and peer pressure. The first and second year data, however, show no differences in drug use between the experimental and control groups. About a third of each group reported illicit drug use (excluding marijuana).[5]

Only a small proportion of each group (about 2 percent) has reported returning to regular heroin use after two years. This low rate of addiction recidivism perhaps reflects the type of ex-addict applying to Wildcat. He has been in treatment successfully for about a year and is motivated to look for work. Wildcat has apparently not further reduced this already low rate of recidivism.

Nevertheless, some differences emerged at the end of the second year in the two groups' involvement in drug treatment programs. About a third of both groups left their drug treatment programs, but 33 percent of controls who quit reenrolled in new ones, as opposed to 22 percent of experimentals who quit. And more experimentals reported they had detoxed from methadone (22 percent) and became drug-free than did controls (16 percent).

---

[5]Self-reported data on drug use are sometimes considered unreliable by the interviewers. Attempts to verify drug use data with drug programs has met with limited success because of concern about confidentiality: the data collected, however, do suggest that sample members underreport drug use.

Table 3. Percentage of Experimental and Control Groups Receiving Direct Public Assistance Stipends and Amount of Stipend

	Post-Wildcat Experimentals N = 95		Controls N = 217	
	Monthly Amount	%	Monthly Amount	%
First Year (monthly stipend)	$186	42	$196	68
Second Year (monthly stipend)	$222	38	$219	60

Alcohol Use

Wildcat supervisors report that drinking is more of a problem among employees than is illicit drug use. At least one third of Wildcatters have a drinking problem. The figure is similar for controls. First and third year results show slightly less daily drinking for experimentals, but this difference washed out during the second year. Alcohol use appears to be related to employment status: among both experimentals and controls, those who have drinking problems are less likely to be employed.

Criminal Activity

During the first six months after entry, fewer experimentals were arrested than controls, but the differences narrowed by the end of the first year and into the second year.[6] In general, a reduction occurs only for those who remain at Wildcat (Table 4). (The proportion of felony and misdemeanor arrests was similar in the first year but in the second year a higher proportion of controls was arrested on felony charges.)

Conviction rates were similar for the two groups, but members of the experimental group were less likely to receive a prison sentence (Table 5). Sentencing appears to be related to employment status; in both groups, convicted participants who had jobs were less likely to receive a prison sentence.

---

[6]New York Police Department arrest records are used as the most reliable and least biased measure of criminal activity. However, self-reported data on hustling and criminal activity parallel the verified arrest data.

Table 4. Percent of Experimentals and Controls Arrested in First and Second Year

	Experimentals N = 258	Controls N = 258
Year Prior	34	37
First Year*	25	31
(1st six months)†	12	19
(2nd six months)	16	17
Second Year	23	22
(1st six months)**	13	13
(2nd six months)	16	12

*x^2 = 2.8, p.c. < .1
†x^2 = 3.8, p.c. < .05
**n.s.

Table 5. Disposition of Arrests (Percent of Arrests, Excluding Pending Cases)

	First Year		Second Year	
	Experimentals N = 53	Controls N = 64	Experimentals N = 66	Controls N = 61
	%	%	%	%
Dismissal	42	41	38	33
Convicted	58	59	62	67
Fine	(4)	(8)	(11)	(7)
Conditional Discharge	(21)	(13)	(11)	(18)
Probation*	(25)	(9)	(15)	(5)
Prison	(9)	(30)	(26)	(38)
	100%	100%	100%	100%
Mean Sentence (months)	4.6 months	8.8 months	4.6 months	13 months

*First year: x^2 = 22.06, p.c. < .01
Second year: n.s.

Experimentals employed at Wildcat had lower arrest rates (.21)[7] than experimentals who were terminated (.56) or graduated (.34). For controls the arrest rate was .43.

---

[7]Arrest rates are per person-year measures that reflect the average number of arrests of a member of a group during a year. Thus a rate of .33 arrests per person-year would mean that an individual would have one in three possibilities of being arrested. Rates rather than percent arrested are used when the time period varies among groups.

To gain a better understanding of whether supported work or employment *per se* affects amount of criminal activity, the proportion of controls arrested who worked in the first year of the study was compared with those who did not work. Twenty-nine percent of those controls who worked were arrested the year prior to the study compared to 39 percent of the controls who did not work. During the year after entering the study 26 percent of the controls who worked during the first year were arrested and 33 percent of the nonworking controls were arrested. These data suggest an association between employment and criminal activity but do not tell whether high criminal activity reduced employment or another factor (such as lack of motivation) caused both arrests and unemployment.

General Living Patterns

It was assumed that if Wildcat affected employment rates, it would also affect other living patterns of its employees. The mobility, health, and education patterns, family arrangements, and schedules of daily life both before and after Wildcat have been compared for experimentals and controls. During the first two years, Wildcat participants were more likely than controls to be financially supporting more than two people,[8] to be living in a stable relationship with another person, and to have children living with them. Although more experimentals than controls were hospitalized during the first year after entering the study, experimentals during the second year were less likely than controls to be hospitalized. (Because the majority of hospitalizations among this group resulted from alcohol problems or violence, less hospitalization is interpreted as a positive adjustment.)

In sum these findings suggest that experimentals were more likely than controls to be seeking a settled life.

COSTS AND BENEFITS: DOES THE INVESTMENT IN WILDCAT PAY OFF?

When it planned Wildcat, the Vera Institute wished to explore not only the issue of employment and its effects on ex-addicts, but also whether it was possible to create a financially sound supported work program. The following analysis therefore focuses on costs and benefits to the taxpayer (rather than the participant). Although the benefits of Wildcat are expected to extend beyond

---

[8]The difference was statistically significant at end of Year One: at end of Year Two the difference had narrowed and was no longer significant.

two years, this analysis is limted to the first two years after entry.[9]

The average annual cost of maintaining an employee in Wildcat is $9,500 and since on the average, a Wildcat employee stays with the program for a year, the taxpayer investment in him is $9,500. This cost is borne by (1) earnings for services provided New York City public and private agencies, (2) diverted welfare funds, and (3) grants from public agencies.

Benefits, not as easily calculated as costs, are divided into two categories: (1) those that result from public services performed by Wildcat employees (e.g., the value of work performed in maintaining police precincts or painting fire stations), and (2) those that result from the rehabilitative effect Wildcat has on its participants (e.g., reduced dependence on welfare and lessened criminal activity).

Services Performed

Two techniques have been used to estimate the value of services provided to New York City's public and private agencies: (1) commerical value of job completed (for instance, the commercial value of tiling a firehouse floor is $1,151, and that of renovating two-family homes is $96,000); and (2) assignment of a value (based on productivity) to the hours an employee works. According to the second method, it has been estimated that a Wildcat clerical employee produces $3.32 worth of services per hour, averaging $6,024 per year; a maintenance worker produces work worth approximately $5 per hour or $9,100 per year. According to these techniques, an average Wildcatter produces $7,000 worth of services per year.

Taxes

Experimentals pay more to the government in income, social security, and sales taxes than do the controls. For income and social security tax estimates, averages were taken from the IRS standard tax schedule. Table 6 illustrates the differences between income levels and taxes paid by experimentals and

---

[9]The data for this analysis are taken from a sample of persons who joined Wildcat between 1972 and 1973. The total costs and benefits of the entire Wildcat population are then estimated by extrapolating the data based on this sample. It was assumed that this sample was representative of the larger population, and data from another more recent sample bear out this assumption. It remains possible, however, that these extrapolations involved some error. Likewise, data on workers' productivity were extrapolated from an examination of 20 job sites randomly selected from the 300 total sites. These findings should thus be viewed as *estimates* rather than firm figures.

**Table 6. Income and Social Security Taxes Paid
by the Average Experimental and Control**

	Experimentals N = 199		Controls N = 217		Difference between Experimentals and Controls
	Mean Income	Mean Tax	Mean Income	Mean Tax	
Year One	$4999	$572	$1118	$ 75	$497
Year Two	$4347	$556	$1854	$120	$436
				Total	$933

controls.[10] The increase over two years in income and social security taxes attributable to Wildcat employment is $933.

An expenditure study of experimentals and controls indicated that experimentals spend 46 percent of their income on taxable goods compared to 41 percent for controls. In the first year, an experimental paid an estimated average of $85 more sales tax than a control. In the second year, the figure dropped to $55 more.

Welfare

A comparison of experimentals and controls (Table 7) shows that there is a decreased dependence on welfare for those who work at Wildcat; and this continues after the experimentals leave Wildcat. (The indirect welfare monies paid to Wildcat for employees' salaries are included in the cost of Wildcat.)

**Table 7. Annual Direct Welfare Monies Received
by the Average Experimental and Control**

	Experimental N = 162	Control N = 179	Difference between Experimentals and Controls
Year One	$406	$1793	$1387
Year Two	$744	$1688	$ 944
		Total	$2331

---

[10]Wildcat employees would be more likely than controls or experimentals not working at Wildcat to pay taxes because Wildcat withholds, but other employers, especially those offering marginal employment, may not withhold as dependably as Wildcat.

Crime-Related Savings

The costs of criminal activity were measured by arrest rates[11] and days incarcerated as a result of convictions (Table 8).[12] It has been estimated that it costs $1,705[13] to process an arrest in New York City. Multiplying arrest rates by the cost per arrest reveals that in Year One, because experimentals were less likely to be arrested than controls, the taxpayer saved $119 per Wildcat employee in criminal processing costs. Experimentals are more likely than controls to be arrested in Year Two, however, resulting in a cost of $68 to the taxpayer. When both years are considered, the net savings to the taxpayer is $51 per Wildcat employee (Table 8).

Table 8. Average Arrest Costs for Experimentals and Controls

	Experimental N = 258	Control N = 258	Difference between Experimentals and Controls
Year One	.36 × $1705 = $614	.43 × $1705 = $733	$119
Year Two	.35 × $1705 = $597	.31 × $1705 = $529	$-68
		Total	$ 51

Incarceration costs have been estimated by the New York City Bureau of the Budget to be $40 per day per prisoner. Since fewer experimentals than controls were sentenced to prison and for shorter time periods (Table 5), the taxpayer realizes savings due to less incarceration among experimentals. Information was not available on the time actually served, and thus, estimates were made according to the length of the sentence. The estimates suggest that supported work saved the taxpayer $645 in the first year and $1,024 in the second year.

Estimated Overall Costs and Benefits

The costs and benefits of Wildcat to the taxpayer for the average employee are summarized in Table 9. For an investment of about $9,500 per employee it is estimated the taxpayer receives $11,984 in two years' benefits yielding a net return of $2,484 or over $1.26 for each dollar invested.

---

[11]Not included is the approximate reduction in crime-related losses to New York residents of $580,000, which would be counted as benefits to "society," but not to the taxpayer.

[12]In 1971-72, the cost per arrest was $1,705 (See Expenditure and Employment Data for the Criminal Justice System, 1971-1972, National Criminal Justice Information and Statistical Service SE-EE No. 4, U.S.G.P.O., 1974).

[13]Table 4 reports percentage of group arrested: however, the cost and benefit data are based on arrests per person-year (see Footnote 7).

Table 9. Costs and Benefits for the Average Wildcat Employee During First Two Years after Entering Wildcat

Costs		Benefits	Yr. 1	Yr. 2
Sources of Funds for Average Wildcat Employee for 12 Months		Estimated Benefits from the Average Wildcat Employee		
Contracts for services performed	$1840	Value of services	$7000	0
Grants from Public Agencies	$5820	Increased Taxes Paid by Employee Income Tax, Sales Tax	$ 497	$ 436
Indirect	$1840	Reductions in Direct Welfare	$1387	$ 944
		Reduced Criminal Activity: Reduced Arrests Reduced Incarceration	$ 119 $ 645	($-68) $1024
	$9500	Total	$9648	$2336
		Benefits Year One and Two = $11,984		

WHAT HAS BEEN LEARNED FROM WILDCAT?

The most important lesson to be drawn from the Wildcat experience is that, with supports, ex-addicts are willing and able to work. Wildcat shows that these difficult to employ persons can, in fact, provide valuable services to New York City. The average Wildcat worker produces about $7,000 worth of services each year, stays in the program for 12 months, and is absent less than one day in ten.

Some of the other lessons are less clear. Does supported work prepare employees for nonsupported work? The absence of a policy requiring employees to leave Wildcat after a given time and the shrinking economy in New York City have contributed to a disappointingly low proportion of employees placed in the open market (14 percent). However, those who have been placed have done well, a finding that indicates that supported work prepares employees to be self-sufficient. But still unanswered is what proportion of the total *could* be self-sufficient and what proportion cannot survive outside supported work environments.

Similarly, determining the rehabilitative value of Wildcat is difficult at this point. The impact of Wildcat upon behavior patterns other than employment has not been powerful. There are no consistently significant differences between experimentals and controls in drug use, criminal activity, and living styles. Is this because Wildcat does not offer more supports to encourage these changes, or is it because employment does not affect non-job-related activities? Was it unrealistically optimistic to believe that offering a person a steady nine-to-five job would change habits built up over a decade or more? Thus far the research has not been able to answer these questions.

Can a supported work program like Wildcat pay off for the taxpayer? The answer to this question relies on the answers to the earlier questions translated into financial terms. The finding that ex-addicts are employable and can be productive means that some of the costs of supported work are reimbursed immediately to the taxpayer in the form of public services. The early results on long term self-sufficiency suggest that the taxpayer is receiving returns both in increased taxes paid by participants and decreased public assistance paid to them. Whether these benefits will be sustained in the third and fourth years is not yet known. But differences between controls' and experimentals' arrest rates in the first six months and in incarceration rates for the first two years result in saving to the taxpayers.

So, in the short run, Wildcat is a good investment. For the dollar the taxpayer invested in 1975, he gets $1.25 during the next two years in services, increased taxes, and reduced welfare and criminal justice costs.

WHAT NEXT?

The promising preliminary results of Wildcat encouraged the Ford Foundation and five federal agencies[14] to establish the Manpower Demonstration Research Corporation (MDRC) to systematically develop and study the supported work concept. In January 1975 MDRC chose 13 sites nationally to test supported work on different types of employees: out-of-school youth, AFDC mothers, ex-alcoholics, and ex-mental patients, as well as ex-addicts and ex-offenders. MDRC supported workers will provide public services but will also expand into the private sector, producing commercially competitive goods and services. MDRC's experience will carry us well beyond what has been learned from Wildcat.

---

[14]U.S. Departments of Labor; Health, Education and Welfare; Housing and Urban Development; National Institute on Drug Abuse; and the Law Enforcement Assistance Administration.

ACKNOWLEDGMENTS

The Vera Institute of Justice has received funds for this research from the National Institute on Drug Abuse and New York City's Addiction Service Agency and Department of Employment.

Index